BODY DEFENSES

BODY DEFENSES

THE MARVELS AND MYSTERIES OF THE IMMUNE SYSTEM

MARILYN DUNLOP

Foreword by Calvin Stiller, M.D.

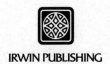

IRWIN PUBLISHING

Canadian Cataloguing in Publication Data

Dunlop, Marilyn, 1928—
  Body defenses

ISBN 0-7725-1565-4

1. Immune response.   2. Immunologic diseases.
I. Title.

RC582.D87 1987   616.07'9   C87-093454-3

Designed by Eskins Stevens Design, Toronto, Canada
Typeset by Century Graphics and Typesetting
Printed in Canada by Webcom Limited

1 2 3 4 5 6 7 8 94 93 92 91 90 89 88 87

Published by Irwin Publishing Inc.

To Duffy and Sammy,
who taught me to value
the search for knowledge.

CONTENTS

FOREWORD

No branch of medicine has grown at a faster pace, both in our understanding of it and in its application to human health, than immunology. When I went to medical school some 20 years ago, the concept of a T and B cell was not part of the curriculum. The possibility of transplants and the concept of auto-immunity were discussed, but without any understanding of their potential application.

A few decades ago, the most common diseases leading to chronic disability and death were caused by infection. Today they are those caused by immune dysfunction. The majority of chronic debilitating diseases — rheumatoid arthritis, multiple sclerosis, juvenile diabetes, chronic lung disease, chronic liver disease, chronic skin diseases, and diseases leading to blindness — are related to auto-immune mechanisms. In short, it is not possible to make sense of current medical literature without some knowledge of the component parts of the immune system.

Today, major breakthroughs in science are announced regularly. Many of them concern immunology itself or the techniques of immunology used to understand fundamental biological processes. The extraordinary advances in transplantation fill the public mind with wonder, and continue to amaze even those in the practice of transplantation, as patients pass from death to life with a success rate of 75 per cent!

In my role as scientist and practitioner–educator, I continue to come up against an interesting combination of ignorance of immunology and its language on the one hand, and a voracious appetite on the other for *intricate* details of the network that makes up the immune system. The most difficult hurdle in explaining to my patients the processes going on inside their bodies, or in giving reasons for medication, is language. Another is communication with members of the medical care team not directly associated with immunology; no easy metaphor has been established to help them understand this extraordinary organization called the immune response.

From time to time there emerges on the horizon of

communicators an individual with the ability to take the complex and intricate and make it understandable. Marilyn Dunlop is such a person and her writings are respected in both the medical and the lay communities for just that. In this book, for which I am honored and delighted to write the Foreword, Dunlop adopts a brilliant metaphor, the *organization of the essential services of a community* — as understandable and accurate a metaphor as I have heard. She is able to take readers into the inner workings of the immune response — examining, for example, a "foreign invader", i.e., a virus — and to help them remember the participants by virtue of their function. Just as clearly, she explains the concepts of auto-immune *disease*, in which the control of these individual workers in the system is lost and an inappropriate attack on the community, in the body, occurs.

Take this book and read it. Absorb yourself in the community metaphor and ask questions. Probe the reason for your medications, or lack of them, and think about how the community network might be rearranged to make the system function better. Much is yet to be known and therefore all questions are valid.

This brilliant work represents a great service to physicians, patients, and the public.

Calvin Stiller, M.D., FRCP(C)

Chief, Multi-Organ Transplant Service,
and Professor of Medicine,
University Hospital and
Robarts Research Institute
London, Ontario

INTRODUCTION

In the past few years, most of us have become aware, suddenly, of a crucial part of the human body called the immune system. It's been brought into sharp focus in the public eye by a disease that scared the daylights out of us, a disease called AIDS, which stands for acquired immune deficiency syndrome.

We'd never heard of AIDS before the 1980s. It had never been seen previously in the western world. But the high death toll among those people who got it, mostly young and healthy beforehand, was terrifying. In modern times we're not accustomed to lethal epidemics. In our lifetimes, almost all infectious diseases have been curable or preventable. Yet here was something that a few doctors termed "a modern day plague."

As we were told by an endless stream of newspaper articles and television reports, AIDS destroys the defense mechanism of the body, called the immune system, leaving the person vulnerable to all sorts of infections and diseases, including cancers. How could that be? If we'd never given much thought to that part of us called the immune system before, we did now. How do our bodies detect these microscopic organisms and generate protection for us? What would it be like to try living in a world laden with invisible enemies such as viruses, bacteria, fungi, and parasites if we had no built-in defenses?

Probably most of us took it for granted that if we caught a common cold or our children came down with childhood diseases, the sickness would run its course and recovery would follow. True, sometimes we were clearly aware there was a fierce war going on inside us. Remember the last time you had the real flu? You felt like a trampled battleground, flat in bed, hurting to the roots of your hair. Yet, once back on our feet, we give little thought to the mechanisms by which we got better.

We might have learned, from reading about transplants of kidneys and hearts, that the patient's body could set up a process of rejection of the new organ. We understood that something within the body knew the tissue was not a natural part of the patient. It seemed astonishing that some other person's heart cells or kidney cells could be recognized as different from our own. Under a microscope, there's no detectable difference. But we considered this simply a medical curiosity, not part of our daily lives.

Today, however, a fascination with the immune system has developed. Physicians tell me that largely because of AIDS, many of their patients are asking "Just what *is* the immune system, doctor?" In our grandparents', or even our parents' generations, doctors would have been unable to give them a clear answer. The immune system was a shadowy thing, despite the fact that for 100 years doctors had been using its presence to good advantage. For example, vaccination, by teaching the immune system to recognize smallpox before it encounters the real thing, has been protecting people from the once-dreaded disease for a century. But for a long time, doctors had no inkling of how the prevention worked.

It has only been in the past 25 years that medical scientists have come to learn the secrets of body defenses. In research laboratories around the world, investigators have been piecing together the explanation. Their remarkable discoveries have disclosed a network of cells as complex as the organization of a big city with its police force, fire-fighters, garbage collectors, teachers, transportation system, libraries, and municipal leaders. Your immune system has, in effect, all those same services at its command.

The riddle of the immune system is not yet solved. Experts in the field would tell you they only know how *little* they know and that they are anticipating that future discoveries will surprise and delight them. Nevertheless, the "little" they know so far is really a great deal and it will enable doctors to work as partners of the immune system in ways never before possible. Some scientists predict that in the next decades, by manipulating the immune system, it will be possible to cure or prevent a number of diseases that today afflict millions of people. Already new kinds of treatments are being devised for arthritis, diabetes, multiple sclerosis, cancer, and allergies, all of which involve the immune system.

This book was written to help answer the questions so many people are asking. Busy doctors don't always have time to explain. It is also intended to help you understand how the immune system is linked to many diseases. If you have a personal interest in certain ones, you can find them by checking the contents list. Information in some of the chapters may help you protect yourself and your families by giving your immune system a leg up, so to speak, with vaccines, nutrition, and other measures. Other chapters covering diseases that cannot yet be prevented may at least offer hope for the future.

Many people today want to take more responsibility for their own health. To do that one needs knowledge and understanding. This layman's guide to the universe of the immune system may help bring you up to date on what medical science has discovered about this marvel within you, a guardian angel that saves your life every day, yet, paradoxically, which can also make you sick.

I hope the book stimulates your sense of wonder about the wisdom of the body and makes you eager to help your immune system keep you healthy.

M.D.

CHAPTER 1

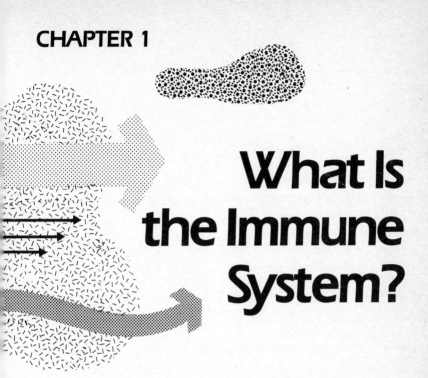

What Is the Immune System?

Unlike your tongue or your heart, which you can locate in your body by sight or feeling, the immune system is not something you can point to and say, "That is it. Right there." It involves a network of tissue, organs, and cells, plus proteins and products the cells create. Constantly, working in harmony, the parts of this network are on the alert for any invader that might gain entry, whether it is breathed in, sneaks through a break in the skin, or finds access to your bloodstream.

Before you were born, as one top Canadian immunologist explains, certain cells of the immune system traveled throughout your body taking note of what was *you*. "I've seen it all," such a cell might say at the end of its travels. "Anything different I notice from here on does not belong and we must attack it." These identifier cells are part of a family of white blood cells called T cells. Originating in bone marrow, they will carry the responsibility for identifying "self" from "non-self" throughout your life.

You also have another family of white cells involved in defense. Doctors call these B cells; they produce antibodies and also originate in bone marrow.

Both these kinds of white cells, which are also called lymphocytes, are produced continuously throughout your life. Each of the cells is equipped with a structure on its surface called a receptor that gives it the ability to recognize one specific substance, one molecule, that does not belong in your body. Not every cell is unique; identical cells — called clones — recognize the same molecule. T cells also carry a receptor by which they distinguish "self." Every person makes a unique protein marker that appears on all cells. It says "me." The T cell receptor reads that message. You have billions of white cells, and clones of cells have an enormous variety of receptors with which they can distinguish tens of millions of different substances.

Cells are instructed how to make their receptors by certain genes they contain. Genes of immune system cells are made of material able to rearrange itself to provide new instructions, hence the great variety of receptors. When a germ — which might be a virus or a bacterium that causes disease — enters your body, some of the cells will have the right receptors to identify it. The alarm goes off and ignites a frenzy of activity, so more troops (white cells) with their weapons are formed to join in the battle. New cells are created by one cell dividing into two identical cells, a process that soon provides battalions of warriors designed to combat the specific germ that has infected you.

You have two basic strategies for defense: doctors call one humoral immunity (humors being body fluids); guards of this system — antibodies — patrol in the bloodstream and lymph. The other is cell-mediated immunity, meaning that a cell (for example, one infected with a virus or one that is not you) is attacked.

Scientists believe the cell-mediated immunity arm of defense is the more primitive and that humoral immunity developed later in evolution. All species of life from highest to lowest have cell-mediated defense, but not all creatures have humoral immunity.

Immunity comes from a Latin word meaning "exempt from," possibly coined by Julius Caesar. For thousands of years simple observation has shown that once a person had a certain infectious disease, a recurrence was unlikely. For example, if you had measles as a child, you are immune to measles for life. Exceptions exist, of course, as you know if you have had a number of colds. But it is true of many contagious diseases.

Nobody had any idea why. But possibly the first people to make use of the observation were the Chinese. They discovered a thousand years ago that persons who had never had smallpox could be prevented from getting it if they inhaled pox crusts taken from patients with the dreaded disease.

But the world would have to wait until almost the middle of this century before scientists gained any real understanding of what the body was doing to protect itself from repeat infections.

The miniscule organisms that cause infectious diseases can't be seen with the naked eye. We sometimes lump them under the general term "germs," but to be specific they are bacteria, viruses, parasites, and varieties of fungus. Bacteria are one-celled organisms that are alive and contain, inside their coats, all the ingredients they require for producing offspring. Our bodies contain some bacteria that are our friends — indeed, we could not survive without them; they produce products we need but cannot manufacture ourselves, including chemicals needed to digest some foods.

But others are enemies, producing toxins that make us sick. They are the causes of cholera, diphtheria, toxic shock syndrome, and typhoid, to name just a few bacterial diseases.

Bacteria can be seen under an ordinary microscope and are usually round or rod-shaped. Viruses, however, are even smaller and can only be seen with an electron microscope, magnified many thousandfold; the palm of your hand, magnified as many times, would seem the size of a big city. It's been said that 10 million viruses could sit on the head of a pin. Unlike bacteria, which are self-contained organisms able to reproduce themselves without help, viruses need a living cell in which to grow. In effect, they take a cell hostage and force it to use its machinery to make thousands of viruses. A virus consists only of genetic material wrapped in a protein coat. Diseases caused by viruses include smallpox, the common cold, rabies, measles, and influenza.

Fungus infections occur most often in the mouth or vagina; a common one is caused by a yeast called candida albicans, which normally inhabits the body but can cause trouble when there is an excess of it. White spots in the mouth, often called thrush, are this kind of fungal infection.

Disease-causing organisms gain access to our bodies by several routes. We may breathe in a common cold virus or take in a cholera bacterium in water. Or the rabies virus might get past our skin if we're bitten by a rabid animal. But whatever the site of entry, the immune system will soon detect the presence of an enemy.

While the whole story of the immune system is not known yet, virtually every day, from a laboratory somewhere in the world, a new tidbit of information is added. It is becoming clear that the immune system is more complicated and far-reaching than ever before suspected. To help us understand, let's begin by meeting the cast of characters playing key roles in our internal daily dramas.

The next few pages may seem as confusing as meeting a lot of new people at a party whose names you can't hope to remember. Don't despair. This isn't intended to test your mental endurance. It is simply a line-up of the immune system components to which you can refer as you read later chapters and want to be reminded of what a B cell or a macrophage is. The contents list at the front of the book is your page guide.

Ready? Then step up and meet:

IMMUNE CELLS

Macrophages

Frequently these large white cells, pronounced mac-ro-fages, the garbage collectors of the body, are the first defenders that a germ or dust particle or other alien invader encounters. They have ruffled surfaces and the amazing ability, in effect, to unzip a piece of their coat and wrap it around an unwanted intruder. They simply engulf and literally chew up with chemicals the foreign particle. Some of them take up residence in specific organs, such as the lungs, spleen, and liver. Others are constantly on patrol in the bloodstream, on the alert for invaders. At the same time, they keep the blood cleansed of aged cells that no longer function and of cell debris.

Their appetites are enormous. They eat an estimated 300 billion defunct red blood cells every day. Without them your blood would become sludge unable to flow. They are constantly at work in the lungs' airways, clearing them of germs or particles of pollutants, engulfing particles of asbestos or silica dust as enthusiastically as living matter. In half an hour, a macrophage can envelop an amount of material half its own size. If a macrophage takes in a particle it cannot chew up, it may carry the particle out of the lung and into the food tube, so the body can get rid of it via the digestive tract.

These refuse collectors also present foreign materials to T cells, bringing into action that line of defense. Macrophages may carry germs or particles to sites in the body where other immune cells gather to show them the invaders and get them to join the fight. When they were first discovered by a Russian scientist, Elie Metchnikoff, in 1882, nobody saw how crucial to life they are. Today we know they play an essential role in both T cell and B cell lines of defense. It is almost certain a person could not survive long without macrophages. No vertebrate has ever been found to exist without them.

They are part of a family of cells called phagocytes (cell eaters). This family also includes cells called granulocytes. Another white blood cell which, like macrophages, shows foreign material to T cells is a dendritic cell. Residing in organs as home guards, they don't patrol in the blood like macrophages. Like spider webs, they have fibers stretched out from the cell body to trap invaders.

But macrophages are the most important of phagocyte cells. When a macrophage swallows an intruder, it breaks down the germ's proteins with enzymes, chemicals that snip them apart in precise ways. The macrophage will then make use of some protein molecules, putting these fragments on display on its outer surface, where they'll be recognized by certain T cells. Such fragments are called antigens. The macrophages also produce a vital substance called interleukin-1. Without it, an immune response cannot take place. It is a signal given to T cells to begin the combat process. As many as 50 compounds are produced by macrophages.

Gradually, scientists are learning what each of these substances is designed to do.

Macrophages start life in the bone marrow. Two Canadian researchers, Dr. Ernest McCulloch and Dr. James Till of the Ontario Cancer Institute in Toronto, were the first to discover that macrophages and their cousins, neutrophils, basophils, and eosinophils (collectively called granulocytes), all originate in bone marrow as the progeny of the same ancestor that doctors call a stem cell. All the cells in your blood, white and red, have a single granddaddy cell, called a multipotential stem cell. Every day you produce millions and millions of new blood cells, all of them crucial to your health, but none more important than the incredible macrophage.

T Cells

These white cells, which doctors also call T lymphocytes, are the bosses of the system. About half to two-thirds of the white cells in the bloodstream of a healthy person are T cells. As young, immature cells, they go off to school. Their classroom is the thymus, a small organ situated just above the heart. It's from the T for thymus they get their name. When you were young, your thymus was larger than it is now. As the years went by, it kept shrinking. But as an adult, you have educated T cells inhabiting various sites of your body. Some cells, which position themselves in strategic locations, have memories. They might be considered your personal historians, able to provide, from their past experience, information your immune system needs.

Some scientists think immature T cells already know what they want to be when they grow up, even before they leave the bone marrow. But so far it isn't known exactly when each particular cell determines which kind of T cell it will be. Yet it is known that if you were born without a thymus, you would lack the T cell line of defense.

At school in the thymus, young T cells learn to follow a career as a special kind of defense worker. Only some graduate — the top of the class, in effect — to give you the best protection your body can muster. These cells go out into the wide world within your body to take up jobs as helper, suppressor, or killer cells.

T cells form the line of defense that attacks cells, going after cells that belong to you but are infected with a virus, for example; or cells that do not belong to you, such as those in a transplanted organ; or cells gone wrong that have turned cancerous. By means of molecules on their surface, called the T cell receptors, they recognize you — self — from what is foreign — non-self. They will attack when they recognize something different, an intruder, along with the "self" marker. For instance, a virus particle along with a self marker tells them that cell is infected and must be destroyed, despite the fact it is a natural part of you. Collectively, T cells can identify an enormous number of potential enemies. As one top immunologist says, "These receptors can recognize just about any substance the universe can present."

Most plentiful of T cells are helper cells. Basically, T helper cells live up to their name. They help other T cells go for the kill; help antibody-producing cells turn on production of antibody; and also help macrophages, enabling them to engulf and destroy invaders. Rather like field commanders, they don't make the kill themselves, but point out the enemy and order the troops to go after it, either by secreting proteins that are messages to other cells, or by directly touching the other cells.

Similar to T helper cells in the way it recognizes a potential enemy is a second branch of the family. This branch is composed of T inducer cells, which bring about the maturation of other T cells, so they can do their jobs, in effect increasing the size of the fighting force.

T cells that destroy infected or foreign cells are called cytotoxic T cells. They're the foot soldiers acting on orders of T helpers. When a cytotoxic T cell sees its specific target, indicating an infection within a cell, it will destroy the cell.

Two other kinds of cells destroy sick cells or alien cells but, strictly speaking, they are not T cells; they are distant cousins. They're called killer cells and natural killer cells. The former are like hatchet men assigned to make a hit; they recognize an enemy once it is covered with antibodies. (Antibodies are described later on.)

The other assassins, natural killer cells, don't need antibodies to recognize their targets. They zero in when a virus-infected cell sends out proteins called interferon. Natural killer cells are the advance troops, fighting the war for the first couple of days while the rest of the defense force mobilizes. These cells are also thought to act as guards on the look-out for cells that have turned malignant. They are different from regular T cells, acting spontaneously without requiring special recognition signals picked up by receptors like other T cells. But, like their cousin Ts, they are part of the cell-mediated line of defense.

Suppressor T cells come into play when the fight is over. They damp down the immune response when danger is past and it is no longer needed. If the immune system were a car, they would be the brakes. They stop the incredibly powerful immune response so it won't hurtle out of control. But in case they shut things down too early, they in turn can be stopped by other cells acting as their supervisors.

You might hear scientists speaking of T4 or T8 cells. T4s are the inducers and the helpers. T8s are the suppressors and the cytotoxic destroyers. They are distinguished from each other by the kind of biochemical marker carried on their surface.

Another member of the cell-mediated defense army is the null cell. Not much was known about it until recently. Now it appears that under certain circumstances, such as malignancy, null cells can be turned into tigers by messages from T helper cells, which make them highly aggressive super killers.

T cells produce chemicals, called lymphokines, that are signals to other immune cells. One signal is called interleukin-2; it is produced after T cells get a message, in the form of interleukin-1, from macrophages. Without interleukin-1, T cells can't make interleukin-2, which is a growth factor, making T cells multiply; it also turns null cells into killers.

T cells secrete a chemical message to macrophages that orders them to stay at the site of a battle. It works like a looped feedback system. Macrophages heed the command "Don't leave." They produce interleukin-1, enabling T cells to produce interleukin-2, which is the trigger for T cell multiplication. As T cells grow in numbers, more messages are produced, recruiting more macrophages to the site. And more macrophages means more interleukin-1, to keep the process going, a quite remarkable circle of communication and cooperation—and all to protect you.

B Cells

These white cells are the key players in the second pathway of defense, the humoral immunity. Like T cells, they originate in the bone marrow, but they don't go to school in the thymus. Their job is to produce antibody and they already know what is expected of them when they leave home. From the marrow they travel to the spleen and lymph nodes to await orders from T helper cells. Like firemen at a fire station or soldiers at a barracks, they move out when and where they are needed, although there are always enough of them in the bloodstream to make up about 15 per cent of blood cells.

A supply of antibodies produced by B cells cruises through blood and lymph all the time. We'll come to them in a minute. First, let's look at the B cells (also called B lymphocytes) that produce them.

Like T cells, each B cell becomes active only in response to one specific target. It is as if that target particle is the key that fits the B cell's motor and starts it up. When T helper cells, the commanding officers of the immune forces, dash into the B cell barracks to report the presence of a particular kind of invader, the B cells that are primed to fight that specific invader are revved up, increasing their numbers dramatically in order to produce many more antibodies.

Overall, B cells can recognize millions of different foreign particles. One cell differs from another in what it recognizes by shuffling certain genes, rather as we switch around the letters of the alphabet to make different words or sentences.

The B cells that produce antibodies are known as plasma cells. Antibodies are poured out into the blood stream, and also appear on the outer coat (membrane) of the B cell where they act as receptors. A receptor is like the keyhole that the molecule — or key — on the germ fits. Other B cells are called memory cells; they perform the task of remembering a particular invader in case others like it ever come again. These memory cells live a long time, whereas other B cells die off after the fight is finished.

ANTIBODIES

The word "antibody" is really a shortened form of anti-foreign body. Also called immunoglobulins, antibodies are specialized proteins that can sometimes knock an invading enemy out of commission themselves. But more commonly, they need the help of the heavier artillery of killer cells and macrophages. They are shaped like the letter Y, with two arms and a leg. The contours of their arms or claws are designed so that each antibody can exactly fit a molecule on the surface of a particular virus or bacterium, in the same way that two pieces of a jigsaw puzzle fit snugly together. As they float through the bloodstream or the lymph or other body fluids, such as saliva, a particular antibody might bump into but ignore a virus not carrying the precise molecule the antibody claws fit. That virus would be some other anti-body's worry.

But when an antibody meets its matching molecule it hangs onto it for dear life. It might meet the molecule floating free in body fluids, or find it on the surface of a macrophage that has already engulfed the organism it came from. To produce antibodies, B cells require the help of T cells, with the whole immune team working in concert. But antibodies alone can halt some infections. For example, an antibody firmly attached to a virus can prevent that virus from getting into a cell so an infection doesn't begin; or antibodies can grab onto toxins produced by bacteria, neutralizing the poison and preventing it from reaching body tissues. Some antibodies recruit special proteins called complement, circulating in the blood, starting up a chemical cascade of reactions that will literally blow the enemy apart.

Antibodies were discovered almost 100 years ago. But until the 1950s, scientists believed all cells in the body made them. With the discovery that they were created only by certain lymphocytes (B cells), intensive research into these cells began, and over the next 10 years researchers learned a great deal about how they work. Much more recently, it was found that they follow the commands of T cells and are turned on by helper T cells and shut off by suppressor T cells.

Five groups of antibody or immunoglobulins are known. Each is commonly known as Ig (short for immuno-globulin) with a letter added.

IgA is the kind primarily found in secretions such as saliva, tears, sputum, sweat; in the digestive tract and respiratory tract; and in vaginal secretions, semen, and breast milk. It is your first line of defense, on duty at the portals to catch a germ before it can enter the inner sanctum of the body. Before a baby is born, no IgA is produced. To give a newborn this kind of protection quickly — and to defend the child against intestinal germs common in infants — breast feeding is important and is one reason mother's milk is more beneficial to a baby than formula.

IgG is the most plentiful kind of antibody circulating in the body. About three-quarter of antibodies in the bloodstream are of this type. It has the ability to cross from mother to child during pregnancy and so provides the baby with the most important form of antibody protection, even before the child is able to produce its own supply.

IgM is a larger antibody than IgG. While an IgG antibody can wiggle its way through the walls of tiny blood vessels and get into other tissue fluids, IgM antibodies, because of their larger size, must stay in the circulation. But these are usually the first kind of antibodies a B cell makes when it goes into action, because IgM is the most effective in bringing into the fray vital substances called complement, which, as mentioned earlier, are powerful weapons with which to blast invaders.

IgD is still pretty much of an enigma. Although it is found on the surface of B cells living in the spleen in quantities 10 times as great as IgM, when a B cell is turned on to produce lots of antibodies, it shuts off production of IgD and begins secreting copious amounts of other kinds of antibodies. Yet IgD is found in a large number of species and as scientists well know, anything that nature preserves in the process of evolution almost certainly has an important role. So far scientists just don't know why IgD is important.

IgE was discovered only about 20 years ago, far more recently than the other immunoglobulins. Scientists believe its purpose is to guard the body against parasites, such as mites and worms. But unlike the other antibodies that protect the body, in many people IgE causes trouble. It is responsible for triggering allergic reactions. IgE is found in low concentrations in the circulation. It also sits on certain cells that contain potent compounds. In people with severe allergies, IgE can bring about life-threatening reactions, including respiratory failure and collapse from shock. The problem is that when it attaches to an allergen (something to which a person is allergic), IgE antibodies that are stuck on cells that store substances such as histamine cause the release of excessive amounts of the compounds. Histamine and other substances pouring out of the cells act on airways and blood vessels, bringing on allergy symptoms. (We'll delve into the story of IgE more deeply in the chapter on allergies.)

Complement

Circulating in the bloodstream are a group of proteins collectively called complement. Until IgM or IgG antibodies latch onto an invader, complement just loafs around; but at that point it moves in. In sequence, the different kinds of complement join in, some of them piling onto the antibody locked to the enemy. At the same time, complement triggers the release of an array of other substances that can knock the stuffing out of the enemy. It can build up fluid inside an infected cell until the cell bursts. It is a powerful and fast method of defense, crucial to the well-being of the body if the invader is a virulent disease organism. Without complement, antibodies cannot destroy bugs that cause infections. They can only put on handcuffs.

Memory Cells

After the battle is over, most of the warriors, both B and T cells, gradually disappear. But a few of both kinds are appointed as permanent watchdogs to guard against that particular kind of enemy, should it ever again try getting a toe-hold in the body. With first exposure, it took the immune system up to seven days to mount a defense. Next time around, thanks to memory cells, it will be ready within hours. You may never even know the germ came back, because it will be zapped so fast there will be no symptoms. While most white cells are relatively short-lived, memory cells are known to live for at least 20 years and some may live as long as you do.

Major Histocompatibility Complex (MHC)

Everything within your body is governed by your genes, which are the codes your cells follow. Scientists call the genes that govern the immune system the major histocompatibility complex, MHC. It is unique in each individual, rather like a molecular fingerprint. The MHC guides a cell in the making of special proteins it will carry on its surface. The particular genes that provide the code for those proteins are known as human leucocyte antigen (HLA) genes. All genes are strung like beads on segments of genetic material called chromosomes; you inherit 23 chromosomes from each parent. The HLA genes are located on the sixth chromosome.

Scientists have isolated many of the HLA genes and given them identifying numbers. They have found there is a close association between some HLA genes and certain diseases. People with a particular HLA gene or pattern of HLA genes appear more susceptible to some ailments. For example, ankylosing spondylitis, a chronic inflammation in the areas where ligaments attach to bone, was determined to be closely linked to one gene named HLA-B27. Almost 90 per cent of people with ankylosing spondylitis have that gene, while in the general population it is found in only about seven per cent. The gene by itself doesn't cause the disease. Healthy people may have it. But if people with that gene meet up with some other factor, perhaps a germ, their body defenses may react in a fashion that starts up a chronic disease. In the chapter on auto-immune diseases, some of the new findings about these genes will be described. Some scientists think the MHC genes dictate the array of substances your T cells can respond to and combat. It is known that in mice, at least, whether or not a particular animal can put up a strong immune battle against a given germ depends on the mouse MHC genes. Even a slight difference in these genes between one species of mice and another can make the difference between a powerful immune response and no response at all.

ANTIGEN

To grasp an understanding of the immune system, we must take into account one more factor. It's called antigen and it is what turns the whole process on. An antigen is something the immune cells recognize. Usually it is a molecule made of protein but it might contain carbohydrate. It is like a name tag or a marker worn by a germ or cell.

Your own cells carry antigens, but your T cells know they are you and ordinarily don't react to them. However, if they "see" your self-antigens in tandem with alien antigens, they know that that cell of the body is infected and must be sacrificed. An antigen is not a whole virus or bacterium. Any given virus may wear a number of these name tags. Virtually anything foreign that gets into your body carries a number of antigens. A measles virus, for example, would not be recognized in its entirety by white cells, but antigens on it would identify it. That gives the immune system an advantage. As we now know, each antibody fits one specific antigen but a lot of different antibodies could fit different antigens on one measles virus. That gives a greater potential for detecting the unwanted visitor.

Antigens come in all shapes and sizes, and it is the shape that is important because it makes an antibody and antigen fit precisely. It is often described like a lock and key. You might wonder why such a precise fit is necessary. Wouldn't it give more protection if all antibodies could fit any antigen? But that could create trouble. Without precise targets, antibodies could inadvertently latch on to self-antigens much more often than they do. An antibody would be more like a master key, fitting all kinds of locks, including those on perfectly normal tissue, and that could play havoc in the body.

The Immune Response

All members of this cast of immune players interact with each other in an endless life and death drama of which we are only occasionally aware. This scene might be going on within you this very minute should, say, a measles virus gain entrance, providing you've never had it before.

Because it is your first exposure, you would not have antibodies circulating in your blood that recognize it right away and fit its antigens. That allows time for the measles virus to force its way into a cell. It will take over that cell and turn it into a miniature factory producing more measles viruses. Eventually the captive cell will burst, releasing hundreds of viruses. But the cell sends out an alarm, by secreting interferon, one of the chemical messages cells use as their language.

That brings natural killer cells to the site to launch the initial attack. On their heels come the macrophages. They engulf viruses, cutting them up and displaying measles antigens, along with the macrophages' own HLA antigens, so T cells can see the problem. Aroused, T helper cells know an invasion has taken place. "Oh ho! We don't want that in here," the helper T cells signal, immediately ordering macrophages to remain in the fight.

Some of the T cells stay and help the macrophages, while others dash off to sound the alarm and bring out killer T cells and B cells with their weapons, antibodies. A flurry of activity follows as all the right kind of B cells and T helper cells multiply frantically. Macrophages latch onto antibodies, keeping them at the war zone, and T helper cells call more macrophages and other cell eaters into action. As antibodies make snug fits with antigens, complement proteins are turned on, pulling the trigger on an array of chemical guns.

Cytotoxic (cell killing) T cells break the membrane covering the infected cell, so contents of the cell, including the viruses, spill out. The viruses quickly fall prey to antibodies and macrophages. Meantime, killer cells of the type that recognize antibody-coated infected cells attach themselves to their targets, setting in motion another chain of events that results in the death of that doomed cell.

Within about a week, the battle reaches its peak and the danger passes. Infected cells have been destroyed, measles antigen has been mopped up by antibodies, and now there is a gradual increase in suppressor T cells to cool things down. Most of the warriors, like old soldiers, fade away. But some memory cells and antibodies to the measles antigens remain on guard in case measles viruses ever show their faces inside you again. It is likely you will never again be made sick by a measles virus.

CELL "LANGUAGE"

All immune cells talk to each other by means of chemicals they produce and release. The first cells at the scene of an infection send out a chemical message through the body, saying where the trouble site is. When they get that message, immune cells begin moving toward the spot. As T helper cells arrive, they release a substance that orders macrophages to stay at the scene. Scientists call it migration inhibition factor. Macrophages release a substance (interleukin-1) that stimulates T cells to manufacture yet another substance called interleukin-2. This substance has powerful effects that make T cells increase in numbers and which turn some of them into killers. Certain T cells bring B cells into action and increase the production of antibodies.

When you have been infected by a germ, you run a fever and your muscles ache because of the action of some of these chemicals. Interleukin-1, produced by macrophages, goes to the brain to raise your temperature. You can blame interleukin-1 for the muscle aches and fatigue that often accompany an infection. So who needs it? you ask. Unfortunately, you do. The catch is that if you didn't make it, your immune system would be shut down and you'd be vulnerable to all sorts of infections. Interleukin-1 is an essential start-up signal to the immune system.

As you mop your burning brow, take comfort in knowing the fever is helping you. Researchers have shown that all immune cells work better at temperatures a little higher than normal. They have found that cats, dogs, lizards, and even fish, sick with infections, have a better chance of survival when they run high temperatures. Interleukin-1 also acts on muscle protein (making muscles ache), so it will break down and can be used for the war effort, providing materials needed by immune cells and for energy.

Doctors call the chemicals that are made by lymphocytes, lymphokines. We'll discuss them more fully in other chapters in connection with particular diseases. Medical science is on the threshold of learning how lymphokines may be used in treatment of diseases ranging from arthritis to cancer. Already scientists know enough to have no doubt they will provide exciting new methods of combating some of mankind's worst ailments.

ORGANS

As you can see, it is the cells themselves that give and take orders, using a language scientists have discovered and partially interpreted in the past 10 years. Unlike the blood circulation system, which depends on an all-important organ, the heart, or the respiratory system, which depends on the lungs, the immune system does not have one chief organ. Organs that are part of the immune system are part of the story, however, and provide the stage on which some of the drama is acted out. They include tonsils, spleen, appendix, lymph nodes, thymus, bone marrow, and clusters of lymphoid tissue in the wall of the intestine called Peyer's patches.

Bone Marrow and Thymus

Bone marrow and thymus are the most important immune system organs. All blood cells, white and red, are produced in the bone marrow, and they all can be traced back to a single forefather cell, an all-purpose stem cell. This stem cell gives rise to more specific, secondary stem cells, which will each produce different families of cells, some having progeny that are red cells, some white cells. Among certain white cells (lymphocytes), some will become B cells, some T cells, as they become altered (differentiate) and follow different pathways to populate your body with the various kinds of blood cells it needs. Thus the bone marrow is the origin of all your immune cells.

Without the thymus, cells destined to become T cells would not become competent at their jobs. The thymus is a grayish organ with two lobes, sitting high in the chest, above the heart. Until the late 1960s, nobody knew what it was for. Researchers trying to figure out its purpose found themselves stymied, because if they removed it from an adult animal nothing seemed to happen. But in the 1960s an American doctor, Robert Good, and other researchers in Australia discovered that if they took out the thymus of a newborn mouse, the consequences were drastic. White cell levels in the blood dropped dramatically and the animals soon lost weight, suffered from diarrhea, and simply wasted away, dying young. The mice could be kept healthy, however, if they were isolated and reared in a germ-free environment, giving researchers their first clue to the role of the thymus in body defense. The thymus plays its crucial role early in life. In humans, it reaches its largest size about the age of puberty. After that it begins to shrink and is largely replaced by fatty tissue. Nevertheless, it is able to keep working, to some extent, until extreme old age.

The thymus produces a number of hormones called thymosin. These hormones are released into the body and help in the cell-mediated immune response. Shrinkage of the thymus may be the result of stress; it may explain, in part, how stress affects the immune system, possibly making people more vulnerable to catching colds or other infections. The thymus has been found to be extremely sensitive to stress hormones produced by the pituitary and adrenal glands. The thymus in experimental animals shrinks within hours of being exposed to these hormones — often called flight or fight hormones.

Spleen

Before birth, blood cells are produced in the spleen, although after birth, bone marrow takes over that job and the spleen becomes a sort of community hall for white cells. A sponge-like, oval organ, about the size of your fist, on your left side behind your lower ribs, the spleen is an ideal spot for white cells to congregate and keep an eye out for intruders. All the blood in your body — about six quarts on average — passes through the spleen every 90 minutes.

Immune cells cluster around the main blood vessel of the spleen. When antigens appear — from a measles virus, for example — macrophages, using tiny structures on their surface called receptors, present them to nearby T cells to be identified, setting off the process described earlier. But while the spleen is a fine watching post, immune cells are also on guard all over the body and so it is not essential to have a spleen to live. People whose spleens have had to be removed, because they were badly damaged in accidents, have a normal life expectancy. However, they are somewhat more vulnerable to infections. In particular, researchers have found that in persons without spleens, levels of T helper cells are not as high as normal. In some fascinating studies at the University of Toronto involving the effects of moderate exercise on immune cells, researchers have found that all kinds of T cells increase during exercise in most healthy people, but that not as many T helper cells are produced in people lacking spleens.

Lymph Nodes

At strategic spots in the lymphatic system, a system that roughly parallels the network of blood vessels, are small, bean-shaped catch basins, somewhat like the filter plants of a municipal water system. These are lymph nodes. As fluids draining from tissue spaces of the body flow through these filters, foreign substances are trapped. Some studies have shown that 99 per cent of bacteria that enter a node never leave it. They are captured there. They'll be dealt with right on the spot by immune cells. Macrophages also carry to nodes foreign particles they have found elsewhere. Ingenious experiments, with colored particles injected into lungs of animals, have revealed macrophages with the particles inside them in nodes near the chest.

Parts of the nodes are densely packed with macrophages and other immune cells, living in little nests. When antigen shows up, the nests become hives of activity as the cells multiply in number, and these cells, along with antibodies, pour out into lymph fluid going through the system.

Tonsils, the appendix, and Peyer's patches on intestinal walls are other locations where antigens are trapped and where white cells encounter them. There is a heavy and constant flow of white cell traffic through all of them, with blood and lymph providing the transportation system on which they ride in ceaseless vigilance.

In all, we begin to understand the wonderful surveillance system within us, designed to ensure that no enemy, no germ that could make us sick, goes undetected for long. Once the invader is spotted, a life and death battle begins. Although we seldom realize it, our own survival is at stake almost daily.

Even a seemingly mild virus infection would be a killer if we had no immune system. A single virus, taking over a cell, would turn it into a factory in which to churn out thousands more viruses. Each of them, in turn, would repeat the take-over of another cell. With no way to stop them, viruses could hold hostage or destroy all the cells of your body. Mankind could not exist without an immune system.

In the next chapter we'll discover what it is like to have an immune system that doesn't work effectively.

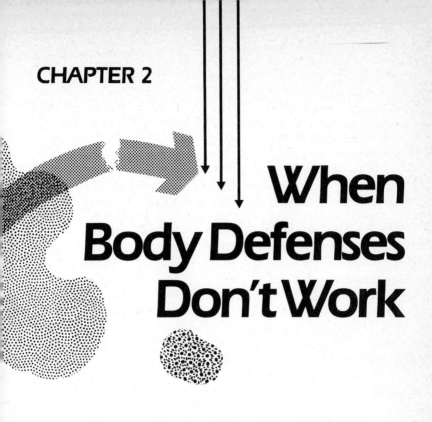

CHAPTER 2

When Body Defenses Don't Work

INHERITED IMMUNE DEFICIENCIES

Long before AIDS began to horrify us, doctors had been seeing patients whose immune systems didn't work. They were children, born that way. The condition was not common and wasn't contagious. For the most part, the public heard little about these patients. One such child, however, caught our attention.

He was known to the world as David — the boy in the bubble. His family name was never made public but when he died in 1984 at age 12, the plight of the little Texas lad had tugged at heartstrings of people everywhere. David had lived his life inside a series of plastic bubbles, their size keeping pace with his growth. He was born with a condition called severe combined immune deficiency syndrome (SCID). Neither the B cell nor the T cell line of his immune system was effective. He was defenseless against the vast array of germs and organisms existing on earth that can cause disease.

David lived as long as he did only because immediately after birth he was put in a germ-free plastic bubble. Throughout his life, until briefly before the end, he breathed germ-free air pumped into his transparent cage. The food he ate was sterilized and there were many kinds of food he could never have. He could never be hugged by his family, never pat a puppy or touch the ordinary things in his home that he could see through the plastic. "He stands out as the clearest example of immune deficiency," his chief physician, Dr. William Shearer of Houston, has said.

David had virtually no T cells and only a few B cells. As discussed in Chapter One, both originate in the bone marrow. Some children like David had been cured by a bone marrow transplant, and the boy's doctors attempted to give him an immune system by transplanting bone marrow from his sister. Tragically, before the transplant could supply him with immune cells, a virus infected David's own scanty B cells, causing them to increase wildly, but without the ability to defend him. Wild, uncontrolled growth of cells is cancer and David developed B cell lymphoma.

The transplant failed; four months later the boy, whose winsome face we had seen many times in newspapers, was dead. But David's legacy to the world was to give doctors new insight into the immune system. From David, we got glimpses of how impossible life would be without a vigorous immune system on guard every minute. Doctors learned that even a sterile environment, like a bubble, could not be made totally free of microscopic life. The human body harbors organisms naturally that are there throughout life. As long as our immune systems are in order, they don't make us sick. Doctors found about 35 such organisms in David's bubble. Although David died as a result of being taken out of his bubble, doctors say some 85 per cent of infections in people lacking a full range of body defenses are caused by organisms — ordinarily harmless hitchhikers — that have inhabited them since birth.

For David, possibly the happiest time of his life was the short period he was free from a bubble and could feel the warmth of his parents' arms around him. With awe and wonder, he touched and stroked objects, able to appreciate for the first time his sense of touch, much as a blind child, given sight, experiences the world in a whole new way.

Some other children with combined immune deficiency disease have had successful bone marrow transplants. More than 15 years ago at the Hospital for Sick Children in Toronto, a baby was cured with a transplant from an older child in the family whose tissue matched closely. Doctors have learned a great deal more about successfully transplanting bone marrow, and today are giving transplants to children like David much earlier. One of the youngest, a little Boston boy named Sean, was given a transplant from his father when he was two weeks old. Gradually Sean acquired a working immune system. At the age of two, he was able to have a dog, play with other children, and eat foods, such as fresh fruits, that can't be sterilized.

An immune deficiency may not be detected right at birth. But Sean's parents knew before he was born that he might have the problem; a brother had died of it at four months of age. As a precaution, Sean was born by Caesarian section to prevent him from encountering, during his birth, any organisms that might be in his mother's birth canal. Apparently a healthy baby of normal weight when he made his appearance, Sean was put in a special sterilized room right away. Tests revealed that the new baby, like the previous child, had the deficiency. Preparations for the bone marrow transplant began.

Usually a child is six or seven months old before an immune system problem shows up. The baby starts to have one infection after another. For the first few months, as in normal babies, antibodies from the mother provide protection. But as maternal antibodies wane, such a child is left defenseless. Fortunately, children are rarely born with defective immune systems.

Not all immune deficiencies can be corrected by a bone marrow transplant. In some children the problem may lie in the thymus gland, so a marrow transplant is not the solution. About eight years ago, at Toronto's Hospital for Sick Children, one of the first children in Canada successfully treated for an immune defect caused by an ineffective thymus gland was given implants of thymus cells. Doctors sometimes call these nurse cells, because they are the first ones that T cells contact when they enter the thymus. The little boy had B cells but not T cells. It took 18 months for the child to develop a T cell line of defense after the implants. But today he is a perfectly normal, healthy youngster.

Severe combined immune deficiency, the defect that afflicted David, accounts for about 20 per cent of cases of children born without normal defenses. Among other disorders that affect only one defense army, about half are defects in production of antibodies. A deficiency in macrophages or other phagocytes makes up about 18 per cent while two per cent are blamed on a problem with complement.

From each type of deficiency, doctors learn a great deal about how the healthy immune system works. If one kind of antibody or cell is lacking, the difference to the patient's health, compared with other children, can be observed. For example, people who don't have detectable levels of IgA antibodies were found to be prone to respiratory allergies, an indication that IgA helps prevent foreign particles from making their way into the airways of the lungs.

Children born with B cell deficiencies were recognized long before doctors knew about T cell problems. The first case reported in medical literature, concerning a child with an immune system disease, was published in 1951. The patient was an eight-year-old boy who, for five years, had had numerous serious infections. It was discovered the lad had no antibodies at all that could be detected in his blood. Furthermore, no antibodies could be found even when he was vaccinated, a fairly clear indication he simply could not make antibodies. At the time, nobody knew there were T cells as well as B cells. As far as was known, antibodies were all there were to the immune system.

Before long, other doctors were reporting patients with the same condition — with no detectable gammaglobulin (antibodies), or at least with very low levels. The names given the conditions were agammaglobulinemia (none) or hypoglobulinemia (low levels). Typically, the problem showed up when a child was about six months old and began to get a series of nasty infections. For the first few months, a baby has protection from antibodies made by the mother during pregnancy, but they gradually disappear and a healthy child becomes able to produce its own. By one year of age, a healthy child has adult levels of the kind of antibody called IgM, and by five to seven years of age, adult levels of IgG. (See Chapter One for a description of the classes of antibodies.)

It is now known that the kind of defect suffered by the eight-year-old boy, agammaglobulinemia, can be caused by a gene a son inherits from his mother. In about one in five such instances, the child has male relatives on his mother's side of the family who also have the syndrome. This indicates that the defect originates with a gene located on the sex chromosome called the X chromosome. Males have only one X chromosome; females have two, providing them with an alternative healthy gene to override a defective one. Hence, agammaglobulinemia occurs only in sons. Studies into the defect showed the problem lies within the B cell itself, occurring in early stages of B cell formation. The children commonly have perfectly normal T cells. But without effective antibodies, they are prone to persistent bacterial and parasitic infections, and they don't build up protection against repeat infections from viruses.

Doctors learned that large and regular injections of antibodies, immunoglobulins, could be lifesavers for these patients. In a dramatic case, one such child with brain inflammation, called encephalitis, which is caused by a virus and can be fatal, recovered completely after a large injection of immunoglobulin. Only recently have immunoglobulin preparations been developed that can be injected into a vein. Previously injected into muscle, they could not readily be given in large enough volume to do the job. For the first time it is possible to give almost normal levels to a patient who cannot produce antibodies of his own.

Immunoglobulins are sometimes used as protective substances for people undergoing treatment of cancer with drugs that suppress their immune systems, or to protect against measles or German measles (rubella) when people exposed to the diseases have not been vaccinated.

Certain people are unable to make the full range of antibodies, although they can produce some. Among them are children, who as a result may have many bacterial infections. Investigating the problem, doctors found these patients had low levels of one kind of antibodies, IgG, but high levels of another, IgM. B cells, circulating in the blood, were making and pouring out large amounts of IgM without apparent cause.

Ordinarily, B cells make IgM first, then move on to production of IgG and IgA. In these patients, the B cells seemed stuck, unable to make the switch.

One of the most common defects, affecting about one in every 700 people, is lack of, or very low levels of, IgA antibodies. Most such people seem quite well; the deficiency is usually only discovered during screening of blood donors. Some of these people do suffer from frequent infections, however, particularly respiratory infections or hay fever. Other parts of the immune system, from macrophages to complement, turned out to be deficient in some people who seemed to be like sitting ducks for germs.

By the 1960s, doctors were recognizing different groups of people whose immune systems didn't work properly. Unlike the children with genetic immune deficiencies, they were not born that way. Their problems resulted from medical advances — drug therapy for cancer, for example. Because cancer drugs are designed to hit cells in the body that are dividing into two to make more cells, a characteristic of tumor cells, the drugs also inadvertently affect normal cells that reproduce frequently. Most immune cells are steadily being renewed, and so are destroyed by cancer drugs. Drugs against leukemias, white blood cell cancer, deliberately destroy white cells. Radiation therapy also hits the armies of defending cells hard. Treatment designed to get rid of a cancer often leaves patients more vulnerable to infection. A quarter of a century ago, many cancer drugs were developed, tested, and shown to prolong life. Yet doctors were dismayed to discover the adverse effects on patients' ability to fight infections. Although the possible benefit of controlling the cancer far outweighed the risk, patients frequently became seriously ill, or died from infections.

At the same time, in the 1960s, kidney transplants had become possible for people whose kidneys were too damaged by disease to recover and do their job of cleansing the body. As transplants became more common, doctors had to learn to walk a tightrope between rejection of the transplant and infection in the patient. The drugs used to prevent rejection were, by intention, substances that damp down the immune system. Rejection occurs when T cells, identifying cells of the new kidney as foreign, bring about an attack on them. Doctors knew that if the transplant was to "take," those T cells had to be stopped. Once again, as in the treatment of cancer, there was a dilemma, for these are the same cells that play a pivotal role in directing the defense teams to fight infectious organisms.

As the numbers of people with immune deficiency from medical treatment increased, the need for better understanding of the immune system became obvious. No longer was the problem confined to the relatively small number of children born with weak defenses. Studies into the immune system had for some years been limping sluggishly along. But with this changed situation, a new impetus was given research designed to pry out the secrets of body defenses.

Throughout the 1970s, research clicked forward. Steadily, a satisfying amount of new information about the complexities of the immune network was being uncovered. But no one anticipated the electrifying stimulus that was to be given to immune system research in the 1980s. Nobody in their wildest dreams glimpsed a portent of what lay just a few years ahead. It was unthinkable that destruction of the immune system could be spread from person to person. But the unthinkable happened and it was named AIDS.

AIDS

Acquired immune deficiency syndrome (AIDS) crept stealthily like a cat burglar into North America. It was here some time before we had any idea how many young lives it would steal. Even after it was detected, most of us paid it little heed. There wasn't much in the news about it, and what was reported made it seem like an exotic, remote disease that only affected people with certain risky lifestyles. Most of us never expected AIDS would touch our lives. Yet within a few years, it was to make an impact on society far greater than the toll of young lives it took. It would bring out the worst — and the best — in millions of people not stricken themselves but forced by AIDS to recognize their own prejudices, becoming aware of the thin veneer of civilization that coats mankind, covering primitive fears that lurk just under the surface.

We witnessed the stark terror of parents marching in angry protest because a child with AIDS was being allowed to attend school, and learned of families and friends ousting patients from their homes, abandoning them with no place to live and no place to die. We felt the shock of discovering that a macho movie hero, Rock Hudson, had contracted the disease as a result of homosexual encounters and was dying. We wept as babies developed the lethal infection from blood transfusions or were born with it because their mothers had AIDS. The AIDS virus infected the soul of society.

But we also saw the unselfish, generous spirit that lies deep within mankind. Doctors and nurses put aside fears for themselves to tend dying AIDS patients before anyone knew what caused the deadly scourge or how it was spread. Strangers opened their homes to deserted AIDS patients. Friends and lovers of the stricken stood by them, disregarding the risk to themselves. Networks were formed of people who volunteered to befriend and support victims of the disease, and thousands gave unstintingly of their talents and time to raise money for research that might find a cure. AIDS not only caused death, it caused hatred, fear, love, anger, altruism, mistrust, forgiveness, bitterness, and compassion.

In 1979, a year and a half before anyone knew AIDS existed, doctors in New York and California began to see something unusual. In both cities, young, previously healthy men were found to have a rare kind of cancer, Kaposi's sarcoma, which got its name from the Hungarian physician Mortiz Kaposi who first described it in 1872. It was odd because in North America it had only been seen in men over the age of 60 with Eastern European or Mediterranean backgrounds, who had inherited a genetic make-up that made them prone to it, or in transplant patients who were taking immune suppressant drugs. Furthermore, the cancer usually only appeared on the skin. In the new young patients, the cancer was more severe and spread through their bodies, occurring in the lining tissue of lymphatic and blood vessels. There was no inherited factor; the patients came from a wide range of racial backgrounds.

By 1981, 21 cases of the sarcoma had been identified, and for a cancer with an incidence of one in 2.5 million people, that was a surprise. At the same time, but quite independently, another strange thing popped up. Five cases of a rare form of pneumonia, previously seen primarily in children with severe combined immune deficiency or in transplant patients taking anti-rejection drugs, were detected in young men who had been healthy beforehand.

Doctors treating these two new groups of patients might never have learned that their patients were the first to be felled by a brand-new disease but for the fact that the Centers for Disease Control (CDC) in Atlanta, Georgia, was the only place to obtain a drug used for patients with incompetent immune systems. In Atlanta, Sandra Ford, a technician who fills orders for rarely used drugs stored by CDC, was puzzled. In one week in April 1981, she had filled five prescriptions for the drug, called pentamidine, from one New York doctor. She confessed later that at the time she thought the doctor should go back to medical school — that he must be making mistakes. But similar orders had arrived from several other Manhattan physicians. Ford wrote a memo to her superiors, listing the cases of the pneumonia and sarcoma among young men. A paper table napkin, taped to an office door at CDC, credits that memo as the tip-off leading to the discovery of AIDS. The impromptu plaque says AIDS was discovered in that room.

About the same time, CDC had been telephoned by two doctors, Michael Gottlieb in Los Angeles, who had treated four patients with Pneumocystis carinii pneumonia (and was later Rock Hudson's physician), and New York skin specialist Alvin Friedman-Kien, who had diagnosed Kaposi's sarcoma in young patients. CDC medical detectives in the field were assigned to do some checking. It was learned that the sick men had one thing in common: they were homosexuals. Beyond that there were no clues to solve the riddle.

By the time the CDC reported on the new syndrome in its weekly bulletin that June, the number of cases of the two rare illnesses had escalated, and of the first 20 patients, eight were dead. Six weeks after Ford wrote the memo, a CDC task force was created to see if the cause of the alarming syndrome could be uncovered. Assigned to head the program was Dr. James Curran, who had earlier coordinated the Centers' venereal disease control division and had also worked closely with clinics for homosexuals in orchestrating the project to develop a hepatitis B vaccine. Because homosexuals are at higher than average risk of hepatitis B, they were a good source of the molecules from blood needed to produce the vaccine.

At the CDC, a headquarters was hurriedly set up, scrunched into basement rooms that had housed laboratory animals. There Dr. Curran began planning the legwork and the hours of in-depth interviews his team members would do. One of the first things they discovered was an inter-connection of sexual contact among the original nine cases in San Francisco. Each of the men had sex with at least one other of the nine. Almost certainly it was a clue. But a clue to what?

Throughout 1981, scant public interest was aroused in the new disease that appeared to affect only homosexuals. Little had been reported about it by the news media. Late in 1981, when I visited Dr. Curran to interview him for the Toronto newspaper where I work, I found an intense, tired and worried-looking man, pinpointing cases on a map of the nation and plotting strategy like a war-time general. He knew the country had already been invaded by an unseen enemy and that it had moved beyond the cities where it caused its first casualties. By that time, almost 200 cases had been uncovered by his investigators, who had contacted physicians working with gay communities across the country. Some men with similar symptoms, it was learned, had died as much as two years before, their deaths unexplained. A typical profile of the patients depicted a gay man who had lived in a fairly fast lane. He had had many sexual partners, hundreds of them perhaps, of whom a number were virtual strangers to him, encountered in gay bars or bath houses. Homosexuals, most of whom prefer to be called gays, had come "out of the closet" in the 1970s. Widespread promiscuity in the decade of the 70s was a phenomenon of the so-called permissive society among both gay and straight (heterosexual) populations.

At that time, no cases had been reported in Canada, although one Canadian living in New York was among the known patients. I was curious, given the rather steady traffic between Toronto and San Francisco and New York, why it had not crossed the border. "It is simply a matter of time," Dr. Curran predicted. "Canada is a year or two behind us."

In February 1982, the first case in Canada was reported.

Although first dubbed the Gay Plague, the disease was coming to be called acquired immune deficiency syndrome and it was also becoming clear not every person affected was a male homosexual. People who used street drugs, injected intravenously, were also showing up with the disease. Some of the infected drug users were women. Like the gay patients, they developed the purplish skin growths of Kaposi's sarcoma, the virulent kind of pneumonia called pneumocystis carinii, and an array of other viral, bacterial, and fungal infections, many of them rarely, if ever, seen in humans. Veterinarians had to be called in to identify some infections previously seen only in animals. It was becoming evident that whatever the culprit was, it was knocking the body defenses of those affected for a loop. Certain drugs became suspect. It was known that some kinds of drugs, including street drugs dubbed poppers, could weaken immune responses. So could a number of common infections, and the idea was put forth that maybe the existence of a multitude of infections cumulatively could be the cause. Gay men, particularly those who often sought casual sexual encounters, were known to be prone to a variety of infections. Yet there had to be something different. Why else had the deadly syndrome not been detected before? It was not something that could go unrecognized, or misdiagnosed, for long. Healthy young men in their 20s and 30s had never before been seen to begin wasting away by the dozens over a matter of months, and dying of rare infections. Half of these patients died of overwhelming infections within a year or so of taking sick.

Still there was virtually no public outcry to spur greater efforts or provide more money to find ways to stop a disease that seemed well on its way to becoming an epidemic. Cases had also appeared in Europe, and while they were far fewer there than in the United States, the numbers were climbing steadily. But members of the general public who had anything at all to say about AIDS were mostly the self-righteous, who claimed it was a well-deserved punishment for sinful lifestyles. Little sympathy was expressed for "gays and junkies" who, some said, had brought the fatal affliction on themselves.

In the summer of 1982, unexplained cases of Kaposi's sarcoma and a brain infection that had been found in a number of gay patients showed up in Haitian refugees in New York and Florida. This was odd, for no Kaposi's sarcoma had been diagnosed in Haiti since 1972 and that single case was in an older person. Even more puzzling, not all the Haitian victims were drug users or homosexuals. But doctors who examined the refugees had no doubt that they had the same syndrome. Later it would be learned that there was nothing special about being Haitian that put a person at higher risk. But it is possible that the virus reached Haiti before it traveled to the U.S., so that more Haitians had been exposed.

The news that stabbed fear into the heart of society came late in the year. AIDS was diagnosed in three children with hemophilia (bleeding disease) who needed regular blood product infusions to help their blood to clot, and in a 20-month-old baby, who had been given many blood trans- fusions at birth. Investigation of the donors whose blood had been used for the baby turned up one with AIDS. The discovery was a horror. AIDS apparently could be spread in blood transfusions and blood products. Were our national blood banks contaminated? And if so, how would we know? Nobody yet knew the cause of AIDS.

In one heartbreaking case, a young man with hemo- philia was infected from a blood transfusion and before symptoms developed passed it on to his wife. She became pregnant, giving birth to a baby who also had AIDS. By that time, other instances in which women had been infected by bisexual partners had also been identified.

From the patterns of disease that were becoming evident, doctors could see that the people at highest risk were the same ones at risk of hepatitis B, which is also spread in blood and other body fluids, by sexual contact, needle injections, and blood transfusions. The cause of hepatitis B is a virus, and medical authorities had become convinced there must be an AIDS virus, too. Yet, while exhaustive tests of homosexual patients' tissues and blood disclosed a lot of viruses, the same viruses also turned up in healthy gay men with no hint of AIDS. The medical investigators also knew that AIDS wreaked its devastation on the immune system by lambasting a particular kind of T cell, called T helper cells, the all- important commanding officers of the whole immune response. That suggested a place to begin looking for an uncommon virus that might be the elusive villain. Maybe it was among a family of viruses known as retroviruses, a sub-species of virus with a different genetic material than most common viruses. Infected cells are forced to make viral genes that are inserted into the cell's genetic material. When the cell reproduces, it passes those viral genes on to its daughter cells. That way, more and more cells become infected. Infected cells are not immediately killed; they become slaves of the virus, unable to perform their own legitimate tasks in the body.

A couple of these viruses, able to infect humans, had already been discovered; one of them, which infected T cells, caused cancer. The two retroviruses had been identified at the U.S. National Institutes of Health in the laboratory of Dr. Robert Gallo. There was also a cat virus, feline leukemia virus, known to infect the animals' T helper cells and destroy the cat defense mechanism. In 1982, two teams — researchers working with Dr. Gallo and a separate group working in a laboratory in Paris at the Pasteur Institute, led by Dr. Luc Montagnier — began searching tissues from AIDS patients for similar viruses. In May 1983, Dr. Montagnier's group reported in a scientific journal that it had collared a suspect. Later that same year, Dr. Gallo's team flushed out a candidate. The French scientists called their virus LAV, lymphadeno-pathy-associated virus. The Americans named theirs HTLV-3, human T cell lymphotropic virus. (Two retroviruses Gallo had identified earlier were HTLV-1 and 2.) It turned that out the American and French viruses were almost identical, differing by only one per cent in their basic chemical structure.

A few months later, a third virus was to join the others, this one discovered in California by Dr. Jay Levy and called ARV for AIDS-related virus. It differs from the other two by some five per cent. Since then, all three variations have been demonstrated to be involved in AIDS. The virus, it was later learned, appears in a number of slightly different guises, because it is able to make alterations in itself.

As researchers studied the virus, they found that when it took over a T helper cell it could reproduce itself a thousand times faster than other kinds of viruses. At first it paralysed the cells; they could not respond to signals that make T cells multiply, nor could they send out signals that mobilize the defense forces. Eventually infected cells die, depleting the potential for counter-attack. Furthermore, blood-forming cells in bone marrow did not replace the lost cells. Scientists also discovered that the virus can infect brain cells, called glial cells, and cells of the brain's lining, as it does T cells. The brains of patients who died showed pockets of dead white tissue. The brain infections affected personality, sometimes causing dementia similar to that seen in patients with Alzheimer's disease. Depression, hysteria, and irrational thinking are also effects on mind and mood that are observed in many AIDS victims. Some patients had severe psychiatric illnesses as the first indication of the disease, even before physical symptoms developed.

The medical profession has defined AIDS precisely, restricting use of the term to cases in which the patient has a life-threatening infection such as the rare pneumonia, or Kaposi's sarcoma, or a profound immune-depression that cannot be otherwise explained. There is good reason for being so restrictive. Many different infections temporarily suppress the immune system and might be mis-diagnosed as AIDS, confusing the picture of the true extent of the new disease. A number of people have developed symptoms such as rampant fungal infections of the mouth and throat that would seem to suggest AIDS but may not be at all. Sometimes they've been said to have pre-AIDS, a diagnosis that could well terrify a patient. But there is no evidence that the symptoms are forerunners of real AIDS.

Furthermore, a second syndrome was detected in the same five-year period in which AIDS was first identified. It involves long-lasting swollen lymph nodes throughout the body and was also seen in young homosexual men. More than a third of AIDS patients had these symptoms six to 18 months before the full-blown disease occurred. Studies that investigated a possible link have found it does not inevitably signal that AIDS will develop. As long term follow-ups of patients continue, it appears that about one in five with the swollen nodes syndrome will go on to develop true AIDS. Although it doesn't help clarify a confusing picture to give different syndromes similar names, this less severe syndrome has come to be called ARC, for AIDS-related complex.

The speed with which the cause of AIDS was discovered was truly remarkable. Scientists could hardly believe it, and indeed many were frankly skeptical that the right virus had been nailed down. But by the end of 1984, the doubts had all but vanished. The virus could readily be isolated from AIDS patients and others in high-risk groups who did not have full-blown AIDS. Injected into chimpanzees, it infects the animals' T cells. Antibodies to the virus were found in virtually all AIDS patients. In effect, AIDS has met all the criteria that science demands as proof of identity of the causative agent of a disease.

Discovery of the virus and antibodies to it didn't help those who already had AIDS. But at least it opened the door for the development of tests to detect antibody. Such tests, now available, are used to screen blood in blood banks for AIDS. The screening test uses parts of AIDS virus antigens to detect antibodies to the virus, by means of an assay commonly known as ELISA (for enzyme-linked immuno-sorbent assay). It is not foolproof, but it will reduce to almost zero the chance of contaminated blood's being used for transfusion. It is not 100 per cent certain, because a person could have become so recently infected there has not been time for antibodies to form. But that risk is slim indeed. Testing of blood donations began quickly in the United States, but took longer to get off the ground in Canada, not beginning until November 1985. By that time more than 300 cases of AIDS had been reported in Canada, but only a very few were the result of transfusions of blood or blood products.

The test to detect antibodies, however, has lifted the lid on a new Pandora's box. When a person with no sign of illness is found to have antibodies, what does it mean? What should that person be told and by whom? In Canada, the person's physician is sent the report, whether the antibodies are detected by Red Cross blood screening or as the result of blood testing done at special laboratories set up to perform such tests on high risk patients at doctors' requests.

The person will be tested again by ELISA, to rule out any possible laboratory error, and that will be followed by a second kind of detection test, called a western blot, a technique that identifies antibodies to virus proteins.

A positive result on all tests means the person has been exposed to the AIDS virus at some time beforehand. It does *not* mean the person will inevitably develop AIDS. Different studies of such people over two to five years have shown that half of them remained free of any symptoms of the disease. One in four developed ARC, the related syndrome that does not necessarily progress to full-blown AIDS. At the same time, presence of AIDS antibodies, in contrast to most other viruses, does not show that a person has been able to mount a defense against the virus and is now immune. Studies have found that a sizeable proportion of people with antibodies also still harbor viruses in their bodies. People with antibodies must be considered as still able to spread the infection. Furthermore, the virus appears to have the ability to hang on for years. From studying patients who got AIDS from transfusions, it is known that the virus must have been in their bodies for as much as five years before it caused obvious disease.

The personal physicians of antibody-positive patients will have to tell them that while they may not develop AIDS, they must consider themselves as possible carriers who could infect sexual partners. Using condoms can decrease the risk. But their doctors will also have to warn them that intimate kissing might be a hazard. The virus has been found in saliva, although no cases are known in which saliva was the sole fluid from which a patient caught AIDS. Nevertheless, doctors have cautioned against deep, open-mouth kissing if one partner has AIDS antibodies or is known to be at high risk of AIDS. They'll be warned not to share razors or toothbrushes with anyone, or any other utensils that could nick, prick, or puncture another person and possibly spread the virus from contaminated blood. Women who want to become pregnant will need special counseling to make them fully aware of the risk of infecting the baby.

For all people who become aware they are potential carriers, AIDS will be a specter that haunts them indefinitely, until much more is learned to determine which people with antibodies are free of virus. Unless you are in one of the high-risk groups, the likelihood you have antibodies is small. But studies have shown that among sexually active homosexuals, needle drug users, hemophiliacs, and women who are sexual partners of AIDS patients, one-third to two-thirds of each group have antibodies. The risk to hemophiliacs is greater than to people receiving blood transfusions because Factor VIII, used to stop bleeding, is made from the pooled blood of thousands of donors, hence increasing the risk.

Among those many donors, one might have had AIDS.

Living in the same household as a patient with AIDS for anybody not a sexual partner has not been shown in North America to be dangerous.

Children, unless infected before birth, have not caught it from their fathers or mothers. Grandmothers or foster mothers who look after babies with AIDS have not developed the disease despite close contact with and cuddling of the infants. Furthermore, no hospital or health care workers have been found who contracted AIDS from looking after patients, with the exception of three who had accidentaly stuck themselves with contaminated instruments. Once outside the body or body fluids, the virus is a weakling, readily destroyed by the kind of precautions that should be taken against any infection — frequent hand-washing, disinfecting with bleach any item contaminated with blood, and careful disposal in a plastic bag of waste such as tissue handkerchiefs or other disposables used by the patient. The virus is killed by ordinary chlorine bleach and by heat. The patient's dishes pose no threat if they are washed in a dishwasher or in hot, soapy water using rubber gloves.

As it became obvious that AIDS was a brand-new disease in North America, the obvious question that arose was where had it come from? As one scientist said, "Viruses certainly don't drop from the sky." For a number of reasons, the finger of suspicion began to point at Central Africa. In Europe, particularly in Belgium, a high percentage of the people with AIDS had come from a Central African country. As well, it had been observed (the observation had gone unheeded at the time) that as early as 1971, young men with Kaposi's sarcoma and other symptoms of AIDS had been seen by doctors in that part of Africa. In the 1960s and 70s, a large number of people had emigrated from Central Africa to Haiti, a possible explanation of why that country's people accounted for so many cases. And blood samples that had been gathered in Africa in 1972 and 1973 and stored as part of a cancer study, taken out of the freezer and tested more than 10 years later, showed that many contained AIDS antibodies.

The pattern of the disease in the African countries of Zaire and Rwanda, however, was different from the west. Almost as many women as men were stricken. It was a disease of heterosexuals as much as homosexuals. Some scientists suggested that would happen in North America, too, as the virus spread out of the homosexual community and into the general population. Others disagreed. They suggested that heterosexuals in Africa had been infected because in that region needles used to give medical injections were likely to be re-used in patient after patient; furthermore tribal customs there such as scarring the skin might account for some of the heterosexual cases.

In Africa, many of the patients were young professional people who had moved to urban areas. Doctors found that promiscuity and sex with prostitutes were common behavior patterns. Epidemiologists (doctors and researchers who trace pathways of diseases) say there are strong indications that AIDS first infected people in rural pockets of Africa who began, in increasing numbers, to move to the cities, bringing the virus with them. They believe that the virus originally made its home in monkeys, probably green monkeys, spreading to humans through bites from the animals.

The findings in Africa have shown scientists that the reason homosexuals have been at greatest risk for AIDS is not because of something inherent in their defense mechanism, but simply that the gay community was the first group in North America in which the virus got a foothold from which it could spread from person to person. Not all researchers, however, are so sure that is the whole reason. In Scotland, large studies of healthy populations found that immune systems of homosexuals among them were different from the rest. There is some evidence that sex hormones are involved and that different levels of such hormones in gay men may make them more vulnerable to infections. In Toronto, investigators at one major hospital have found homosexuals can have unusual antibodies that attack their own immune cells, and they believe these antibodies develop in response to sperm.

Four years after the first few cases of the bizarre new disease were seen, more than 13,000 people in the U.S. had been diagnosed and almost half of them had died. But for much of the population, it was the disclosure of AIDS in Rock Hudson, then appearing in the popular television show "Dynasty," that made the enormity of the disease hit home. This was a person people felt they knew, not a faceless statistic. The movie star, then 59, had made 62 films, co-starring with many top actresses before switching to television's widely watched "McMillan and Wife." He had discovered that he had the disease in mid-1984 but the diagnosis was kept secret until, in July 1985, the six-foot-four actor flew to Paris hoping to be treated with an experimental drug developed at the Pasteur Institute.

But by the time he got there his condition was too poor to make him a candidate for an attempt at therapy with the drug known as HPA 23. He chartered an Air France 747, at a cost of $250,000, and flew home. In October, the star, whose real name was Roy Scherer Jr., died at his Beverley Hills home.

It no longer mattered that the public knew of his homosexuality, kept hidden for so long to preserve his he-man image. A month before he died, Hollywood had turned on the full force of its glamor for a charity gala in his honor to raise $1-million for the Los Angeles AIDS project. Among those with messages for the dazzling crowd urging greater efforts to combat the new killer was Rock Hudson's former acting colleague, U.S. President Ronald Reagan. Patients with AIDS felt a new glimmer of hope that even greater effort would be put into finding a way to beat the killer disease. "We knew that eventually some famous person would develop AIDS," said one Toronto man with the syndrome. "We didn't know who it would be. We'll have to wait and see if any good comes out of it for the rest of us."

While medical scientists repeatedly said AIDS couldn't be caught by casual contact — shaking hands with a patient, working in the same office, eating in the same restaurant, or sharing a communion cup at church — it was obvious that many people remained doubtful. In Manhattan, at the trial of a 34-year-old AIDS patient charged with murder, court officers wore surgical masks and gloves. In Indiana, a grade seven student, barred from the classroom, was obliged to keep up with lessons by a telephone hook-up to the school. The boy, a 13-year-old hemophiliac, had got AIDS from a transfusion. Parents of other children threatened to sue if the boy was allowed in the school. Two years later, in 1986, a court ordered the school to allow him to return to class. It complied, but it provided him with a separate washroom, required him to use disposable dishes in the cafeteria, and would not permit him to take classes in physical education.

In Queens, New York, a thousand people protested a city plan to place three AIDS patients in a nursing home. One of the marchers shouted angrily, "They will be walking in our streets." In a prison, authorities said guards were being terrorized by prisoners with AIDS who were spitting at them. AIDS, it was said, had become the very symbol of Death abroad in the land, and public reaction was described as a medieval *danse macabre*.

New coals to add to the fire of fear kept appearing. In Australia, four women caught AIDS as a result of artificial insemination at an infertility clinic. During 1982, each had received sperm from the same donor but none had become pregnant at that time. Medical authorities said sperm donors and donors of organs for transplants should be tested for antibodies to AIDS in the same way as blood donors. No reports of AIDS resulting from transplants have been published, and the possibility of a donor's going undetected now is low; nevertheless, worry is increased for people awaiting transplants.

There was also reason for alarm in another group of people. A private clinic in Freeport, Grand Bahama Island, had for several years been treating cancer patients with proteins from human blood. Patients were given vials of the material to take home to continue the treatment themselves. Eighteen such vials, given to two patients, were tested in the U.S. and six showed positive for AIDS antibodies. The Bahamian ministry of health ordered the clinic closed. Subsequently, AIDS virus was cultured from one of the samples by technicians at the Centers for Disease Control. The samples also contained hepatitis B particles. Among the Canadians and Americans who had been treated at the clinic was a U.S. state governor. The agony for him and the others is the prolonged uncertainty. If any of them has been infected it could be some years before the virus, hiding itself in their bodies, makes itself known.

News from the research laboratories wasn't encouraging, either. Vaccines would not be easy to devise. The virus seemed able to thumb its nose at scientists. It could change its outer coat, and that could mean one vaccine would not work against all the variations. Even if some part of the virus remained constant, there was no guarantee that the antibodies formed against it by the body would be effective as virus killers. From the cat leukemia virus, a different but related germ, scientists know that even a "killed" virus (one treated with chemicals or heat so that it is unable to reproduce) in vaccine could cause disease. Before it enters a T cell, the cat virus produces poison that disarms the T cell, making it unable to give orders for immune defense before it is captured by the virus. The scientists found that this poison was produced by the virus even when it had been "killed." Kittens, vaccinated with killed virus vaccine, became very sick. But scientists outwitted the cat virus and developed a vaccine that effectively protects cats, immunizing them against both virus and viral poison. It took 10 years, but it does offer hope that a vaccine for humans is possible.

Several centers have teams hard at work competing, through different approaches, to be the first to produce an AIDS vaccine. At one center, in Philadelphia, antibodies obtained from the blood of women who have given birth to babies with AIDS but who have not become sick themselves are being used as a possible model from which to create other antibodies. One problem to be overcome is the fact that while AIDS patients make antibodies against the virus, the antibodies are ineffective. Even those who are convinced a vaccine will ultimately be a reality, however, say it will take at least until 1990.

Vaccines, of course, won't help those who already have AIDS or the related syndrome, ARC. Doctors have become adept at treating the bouts of repeated infections with anti-microbic agents and anti-fungal drugs, and they've looked everywhere for new treatment candidates. For example, an anti-malaria drug that was used with some success in an orphanage in Iran, where there was an outbreak of Pneumocystis carinii pneumonia, is being tried in AIDS patients who suffer repeated bouts of the pneumonia. In Florida, another drug called AL 721, is under study. It represents a whole new method of attack, stripping cholesterol out of the virus coat or outer membrane so it can't push its way into healthy white cells. Natural body substances, interferon and interleukin-2, which are types of chemical messages immune cells use to talk to each other, have been injected in patients in several studies. In AIDS patients, an abnormal kind of interferon has been observed. Doctors theorized that normal interferon might be useful. Interferon is produced when there is a virus infection; it acts as a sort of chemical Paul Revere, warning cells not yet infected to defend themselves. It has been found to get natural killer cells marching to battle. Interleukin-2 is material secreted by T helper cells; it has been found to turn another kind of white cell into a roving killer cell.

One startling method of treatment, attempted first in France, is to use a drug, cyclosporine A, that prevents the rejection of transplanted organs. It sounded ridiculous at first, because the drug suppresses the immune system, acting on the same cells that the AIDS virus infects. Treating an immune suppression disease with an immune suppression drug appeared to make no sense at all. But scientists have reason to believe that the immune system is aiding and abetting the virus. Immune cells attack infected T cells, possibly releasing chemical messages that order the destruction of more T cells than would be killed by the viruses alone. The drug interferes with those messages. It was tested in three Canadian cities as well as in some American centers.

The tests showed within a short time that while cyclosporine A did not help AIDS patients — it made them worse or speeded death — it did bring dramatic improvement in those with swollen lymph nodes and AIDS-related complex (ARC) whose T helper cells had not yet been depleted. Under its influence, swollen nodes shrink, fevers abate, and the numbers of T helper cells and T suppressor cells, badly out of balance, revert to normal ratios. In effect, the drug prevents a patient's T cells from attacking fellow T cells. One Canadian researcher says that ARC, or pre-AIDS, is in fact an autoimmune disease in which T helper cells are destroyed by other T cells. It is, in a sense, mutiny; the fighters turn against their commanders. From the perspective of the virus, it is a clever piece of sabotage. Without commanders, defense forces flounder and the viruses have a field day. By the time AIDS develops, it is too late to rescue the commanders. The drug may work well if given prior to AIDS.

Yet another treatment takes advantage of the peculiar genes of the virus. They are different from the genes of the majority of viruses in that the virus cannot use them directly to make more viruses. It must first make a copy of its genes using material from the cell it has infected. Researchers are feeding the virus some phony building blocks. They make defective genes that don't work when the virus tries to multiply. One drug that does this is called dideoxynucleoside. In early tests, some patients were reported to have improved.

To copy its genes, the AIDS virus needs a special enzyme called reverse transcriptase. The enzyme, carried by the virus, enables the virus to convert its single-stranded genes — RNA — into double-stranded ones — DNA — so they will work like an infected cell's own genes. Scientists are looking for drugs that will interfere with the action of the enzyme. Bone marrow transplants and transfusions of healthy lymphocytes are other methods under consideration.

Every rumor of a promising treatment brings a clamor from AIDS patients desperate to try anything that might save their lives. For scientists, the result has been a many-sided ethical dilemma: Is it ethical to withhold drugs of unknown value from patients? Doctors are not accustomed to giving drugs that could easily do patients more harm than good, when there is no way of knowing the outcome. Ordinarily, they test new drugs on a very few people to determine the safety. At that stage, it is not considered ethical to use a new drug widely. Yet just a whiff of news that some substance might fight AIDS, and hundreds of dying people beg for it. Is it ethical to refuse them? No person with AIDS is expected to live for many years. In scientific studies, a new drug is tested against a placebo (a fake pill that looks like the real thing). Some patients get the real thing, some the dummy, without knowing which is which. Doctors can thus measure the new drug's effectiveness. Is it ethical to assign a number of AIDS patients to a placebo group? Scientists are struggling for answers.

The dilemma became acute when tests with one experimental drug, Azidothymidine (AZT), seemed to be prolonging life in AIDS patients who had suffered a bout of Pneumocystis carinii pneumonia. It is not a cure. But among 145 patients given AZT in clinical trials at a dozen medical centers, starting in February, only one had died by September, whereas 16 of 137 control patients — given dummy pills — died in the same period. The drug manufacturer, Burroughs Wellcome Co., called an early halt to the trial and gave AZT to all patients in the trial. In the United States, a national hot line for AZT inquiries was provided and was swamped with calls. A supply of the drug was also made available for a number of Canadian patients. AZT intrudes on the enzyme reverse transcriptase, causing errors in gene manufacture.

Because AIDS patients have also been found to be suffering from a malfunction of the adrenal gland and so lack certain hormones, some patients have been given replacement hormones to relieve the symptoms that add to their misery, such as nausea, dizziness, and fever. In still other studies, several anti-virus drugs have been found to have an effect on the AIDS virus, at least in the laboratory. One being tried in patients is called isoprinosine, first used in Europe to stimulate the immune systems of herpes patients. At several centers, a cooperative study of the drug ribavirin is under way; this drug is used to treat diseases caused by some respiratory viruses, including influenza A, and to treat Lassa fever.

But early promises are not always kept. Another drug that seemed to offer hope was suramin, previously used in parasite infections including African sleeping sickness. It looked promising in cell cultures in the laboratory, and even in one patient, but it proved far too toxic and didn't stop the viruses from multiplying. In Israel, a 13-year-old boy was the first to be treated with hormones from the thymus gland of calves, with partial success.

Nobody suggests any of the drugs known so far are a cure for the underlying disease. Only the immune system itself, when it is healthy and vigorous, knows how to beat the vile virus. Doctors know that the immune system can defeat it; not all people infected with the virus get sick. In Edinburgh, Scotland, where 33 hemophiliacs were given blood-clotting factor that turned out to be tainted with AIDS, 15 became infected and the others remained disease-free. Studies had been done beforehand on the patients' immune systems, and it could be seen later that the 15 who got AIDS had had low levels of protective white blood cells before the infection. Some experts suggest that the virus, much as lions prey on the weakest of plains animals in a herd, preys on people whose immune systems are already more feeble than normal. Researchers may find new leads to treatment from people whose immune systems have won out.

While so far the pursuit of weapons against AIDS has produced nothing to cause great rejoicing, all is not gloom and doom for those people who must take the risk of getting AIDS from blood products. In both Canada and the U.S., two in 1,000 hemophiliacs (there are 1,500 of them in Canada) have developed AIDS from contaminated blood products. On the horizon is a synthetic clotting factor for these patients, produced by genetic engineering and precluding the need to use products from human blood plasma. The gene that tells the human body to make the clotting substance, called Factor VIII, is one of the largest genes known so far, and reconstructing it artificially has been hailed as a remarkable achievement. Meantime, heat treatment of blood products has also been found to destroy the virus.

It has also become clear that a prudent lifestyle, foregoing promiscuity or use of injectable drugs, is the best protection possible against AIDS. Both in North America, where the majority of AIDS patients are homosexual, and in Africa, where they are heterosexual, it was learned that the risk was greatest in those with many different sex partners. In general, doctors advise people to avoid having multiple and/or anonymous sex partners.

The virus spreads more readily from men to women or men to men than from women to men. But it is a two-way street. Some researchers have suggested that anal intercourse increases the risk of infection because of the likelihood of small rips in the tissue, giving the virus access to the bloodstream. The vagina is much less fragile tissue than the anus and rectum and is designed to withstand sexual intercourse without ripping.

A study in Australia suggests there may be symptoms anywhere from a few days to two months after a person is first infected with the virus. It found that 11 out of 12 men had had a mononucleosis-like illness around the time of the initial exposure. They had fever, night sweats, nausea, loss of appetite, joint pains, sore throat, swollen glands, or rashes that lasted from three days to two weeks. But since AIDS can show up so long after the initial infection, the time a person caught the virus may be impossible to determine. The Centers for Disease Control have reported cases resulting from exposure to the virus seven years earlier. Doctors fear that there are many infected people who don't know they have the AIDS virus and will, quite unintentionally, continue to spread it.

After five years, from 1981 to the last quarter of 1986, the CDC had been notified of more than 23,000 patients. Canada had 645 cases. In the U.S., 90 per cent of patients are between the ages of 20 and 49. More than half had died, including seven of every 10 who had been diagnosed before 1984. Ninety-three per cent are men and 70 per cent homosexuals or bisexuals. Among infected women, about half of the cases were the result of using contaminated drug needles. In general, the experts predict AIDS will not sweep through the heterosexual population as fast as it did the gay community. The CDC listed 1,100 cases in 1986 that it classified as heterosexually transmitted; it predicts there will be 7,000 such cases in 1991, among a predicted total number of 270,000 cases.

But some scientists warn that AIDS is already moving into the general population on this continent as prostitutes, who inject drugs or catch AIDS from bisexual partners, infect straight men. As in all sexually transmitted diseases, promiscuity increases the risk of contracting AIDS. As mentioned, doctors say that the virus does not spread as easily from females to males as from males to females. But as one eminent physician has put it, "It is a great time to be monogamous."

By early 1986, AIDS had cost the United States more than $6-billion in medical bills and lost income, according to a study by the CDC. A typical medical bill for a patient was $147,000. The emotional cost was incalculable.

CHAPTER 3

Auto-Immune Diseases: The Wrong Target

In 1976, at Fort Dix military base in New Jersey, a soldier died of influenza. When medical scientists analyzed the virus with which he had been stricken, it appeared to be one that caused swine flu, the same kind of killer germ that had swept disastrously through the world in 1918. (We'll return to that flu epidemic later in the section on influenza in Chapter Eleven.) The medical scientists pushed the panic button. While their intentions were noble, the chain of events that followed harmed many Americans, cost hundreds of millions of dollars, and to some extent shook public faith in doctors. But it also provided proof, for the first time, that a virus can trigger cells of the immune system into mistaking friend for foe and attacking natural tissues in the body.

It all began when, after an investigation into the cause of an outbreak of illness at the base, the alarm went up at the U.S. Centers for Disease Control in Atlanta, Georgia, that a dreadful variety of flu virus had once again made an appearance. Doctors there envisioned a catastrophe with millions of people sick and many deaths. Only mass inoculation of the public to protect them from swine flu could prevent a national disaster, they said. Within a short time, the American government had put out $135-million to protect people with vaccine and 100 million people in America were given shots.

But the flu epidemic didn't materialize. Instead, a lot of people who got the vaccine developed a form of paralysis called Guillain-Barre syndrome. Subsequently, millions of dollars were paid in damages to these people. Canada escaped a similar scene, not because we were any wiser and recognized the alarm was unfounded, but simply because we were unprepared. We didn't have the vaccine or large-scale vaccine-making facilities that could be geared up in time to produce it. Canada had always relied on the U.S. to be its supplier of many pharmaceutical products, but in this case the U.S. believed it needed all the vaccine it could make for itself. North of the border, the fiasco was limited to political finger-pointing and outrage over why Canada was not self-sufficient in producing products to safeguard the public health.

It had long been suspected that there was a virus connection with Guillain-Barre syndrome. Typically, it develops several weeks after a viral infection. But because mild virus infections are so common, there had never been any proof. The syndrome occurs in only one or two of every 100,000 people. But among Americans who were vaccinated, the incidence was 10 to 20 times that high.

The syndrome begins as muscle weakness first in the legs, then moving up to the body. In severe cases it affects respiratory muscles, leading to respiratory failure. It affects nerves controlling muscles, rather than muscle tissue itself. Usually it reaches its worst peak within a month and then the patient begins to recover.

Studies of patients with the syndrome revealed that myelin, the insulating sheath that covers nerves, was being attacked and damaged by T cells. In Guillain-Barre syndrome it is the nerves in the legs, chest, and arms that are affected, rather than the central nervous system of the spinal cord and brain, as occurs in multiple sclerosis. For the first time beyond a shadow of a doubt, it could be seen that a virus, the one used to make the vaccine, had led the T cells astray, misdirecting the home troops. When that happens, doctors call it an auto-immune disease. (Auto means self in medicine, the same as it does in autobiography.)

The syndrome is only one of a number of diseases that doctors have reason to believe are auto-immune diseases. Multiple sclerosis, arthritis, diabetes, lupus, and a variety of other ailments that affect large segments of the population, are among them. While until now treatments to help overcome symptoms have been useful, none of them gets at the root of the trouble. The causes of the diseases were, and still are, unknown. But over the past 10 years, evidence has been accumulating that these diseases occur when something has turned cells of the immune system toward the wrong target so that they begin, in effect, waging civil war. What that "something" is, in most diseases, has not yet been firmly nailed down. Viruses and other infectious organisms, of course, are high on the suspect list. But the jury is still out and there is no verdict yet on whether germs are the guilty parties in any of these diseases.

If germs turn out to be involved, safe vaccines to prevent many disabling conditions might be possible. That is one hope for the future. But even today the recognition that these conditions are almost certainly auto-immune diseases has made possible a brand-new approach to treatment and may have a profound effect on strategies to prevent them.

To help us gain better understanding of the new findings, we'll look at a number of such diseases individually.

MULTIPLE SCLEROSIS

The most common central nervous system disease in young Canadians and Americans, multiple sclerosis is a condition in which myelin in the brain and spinal cord is damaged, interfering with transmission of messages from the brain. Its impact varies from patient to patient, but it can disrupt the ability to walk, see, speak, or retain balance. Myelin is like the insulation on an electrical cord. If it is frayed, the electrical currents are short-circuited. Symptoms may come and go mysteriously — doctors call the waxing and waning of symptoms remissions and recurrences — but typically it worsens over time until there are no more remissions. MS has been around for a long time. It was first described in France in 1877, although making a definitive diagnosis even today is usually not easy.

The disease is much more common in temperate countries like Canada than in the tropics, with some 30 to 90 cases per 100,000 people here compared with three per 100,000 in places farther south, like New Orleans. It is rare in some countries such as Japan, yet very familiar in northern Saskatchewan and the Shetland Islands. Usually it hits people between the ages of 20 and 40.

In recent years, scientists have discovered that the damage to myelin is being done at least initially by macrophages. Part of their job is to present molecules of foreign material (antigens) to T cells, which "see" unwanted invaders. When a T cell recognizes an antigen, it becomes active and orders up combat troops. Wherever that antigen is spotted becomes a war zone.

Combat troops apparently have been called to the central nervous system of people with MS. Doctors can find certain kinds of T cells there in unusually high numbers. There are different subsets of T cells, and researchers have found in spinal fluid and brains of people with MS that the kinds of cells present in large numbers are primarily cytotoxic (killer) T cells. It's clear that they've moved there for some reason, but what has drawn them remains a puzzle. It isn't yet known why macrophages begin to attack myelin, nor what the antigen is that they present to T cells and which is being recognized as an enemy.

Researchers found a substance called myelin-basic protein, which they thought might be the antigen that was mistaken for a foe. Myelin is made of a double layer of fatty tissue with protein imbedded in it. They found that white cells from some (but not all) MS patients will react to myelin-basic protein as if it were foreign. Yet studies have found that normal blood cells from healthy people can also react the same way. Why, then, don't they develop MS? Clearly, some other factor is at work and it may lie in the genes. If myelin-basic protein is injected into mice, some species will show a fierce immune response and will develop a disease that is much like MS. In other species, no disease develops. It would seem that some mice and some people are more susceptible. Their genetic make-up may be the reason that they are at greater risk.

A genetic connection fits in with the fact that there are larger numbers of cases among people with Northern European backgrounds who have a common ancestry, while other races have low numbers of cases. Yet the picture is confusing, because an increase in MS is being noted in Israel among people of Middle-Eastern descent who should be, like their ancestors, at low risk. This changing pattern may lend weight to the belief that a virus is the culprit. Some experts think that as Israel has developed as a nation, more of its inhabitants are middle class people living in communities with good sanitation whose children generally don't get certain contagious diseases at an early age and who therefore don't build up antibodies to various diseases. Catching such diseases after early childhood can mean people get more severe cases. That was true of polio, a viral disease that did its greatest damage among middle class North American families.

Late in 1985, a team of scientists from one Swedish and three American research centers reported that they had discovered a possible connection between MS and a previously unknown virus. The report spread great fear among MS patients. They got the mistaken idea that this unknown virus was the AIDS virus. It is not. It is a remote cousin of the virus that causes AIDS — a type of virus called a retrovirus. The genes of these viruses are made of a different kind of material from most other viral genes. They are relatively common in animal species but so far only four are known to infect mankind. The team found what might be called footprints of the new virus in cerebrospinal fluid from 52 patients in Sweden and in Key West, Florida, where in recent years an unexpected cluster of MS cases has occurred. They did not find traces of the new virus in 100 healthy people or in 17 with other neurological diseases. The scientists also found higher levels of antibodies to retroviruses in the blood of 60 per cent of MS patients. In one case, in which antibody levels were measured over several months, the scientists saw a rise in these antibodies coincide with an acute recurrence of MS. The findings, while fascinating, provide no proof the newly identified virus is the cause of MS. Many doctors believe the cause is probably an interplay among a number of factors, one of which could be a virus, but perhaps not always the same one in all MS patients.

In any case, researchers are beginning to see a lot of unusual things going on in immune cells of MS patients. They have learned that during an acute attack of MS, the number of suppressor T cells — the cells that call a halt to an immune battle — show a marked decline in activity. There are fewer of these cells in the blood. Chicago researchers have discovered that suppressor cells have proteins on them similar to proteins found on cells that make myelin. They suggest that during an attack, whatever is destroying myelin may also be destroying suppressor cells, the very cells that could stop the attack.

In Boston, investigators have also found in the blood and spinal fluid of patients some T cells that are active when ordinarily such cells would be resting. T cells remain at rest most of the time, until they are shown antigens that they are primed to recognize. Each cell (or more accurately each clone of cells, which are all identical) sees only one particular antigen. Researchers are trying to find out which particular antigen is turning these T cells on and why they are not turned off again. Scientists use experiments that investigate cells in the laboratory and in animals to ask questions such as these: Is there some flaw in the T cell receptors of MS patients that makes them act wrong-headedly? Is the problem that they do not know when to quit because suppressor cells have gone missing in action? Are there abnormal proteins in the myelin of these patients? The different patterns of T cells in patients as compared with healthy people has led some doctors to think the disease arises because of a defect in the immune system itself. It may be that present in perfectly healthy people are T cells that might attack the body if they weren't kept firmly in check by suppressor cells.

Other scientists are convinced the self-attack process begins with a virus. They have several reasons. Where a person lives in childhood is one clue. If someone moves before the age of 15 to a different region of the world, his or her chances of getting MS will change in accordance with the incidence in the new region, becoming higher or lower accordingly. After the age of 15, a move will make no difference. That suggests to scientists that an infectious organism of childhood might be the culprit. (The incidence of some other diseases, such as cancer, also changes in populations that move to new countries, but there is no age cut-off. For example, among the Japanese who moved to British Columbia, Canada, the rate of stomach cancer decreased and the rate of colon cancer increased, bringing the incidence of both close to the rates of other Canadians. A change in diet is believed to be the cause. But no diet factor has been found to be involved in MS.)

Measles has come under particular suspicion, and many studies have shown high levels of antibodies formed against measles in MS patients.

The measles virus is known to be able to infect central nervous system tissue, causing brain inflammation, which is the key reason it is not a trivial disease. Some investigators have suggested that people who get measles at a later age might never get rid of the virus entirely, and that MS is the result of a persistent immune cell attempt to pry it out. A public health study in Los Angeles found that as far as childhood diseases went, the only difference between 88 MS patients and 88 healthy contemporaries was that the MS group consistently reported having measles at an older than average age.

Strengthening the case against measles is the finding of other California researchers that a stretch of measles virus protein (the particular sequence of building blocks, amino acids, of which proteins are formed) is identical to myelin protein. The virus might scoop up the myelin protein to use in reproducing itself, leading T cells to see myelin as virus.

If measles virus is the trigger, it's possible that there will be a great decline in MS, as widespread vaccination of children eventually wipes out measles epidemics.

Other researchers are still casting a beady eye on the distemper virus that can infect and kill dogs. It was first held up as a candidate because MS, which had been unknown on the Faroe Islands, midway between the north of Scotland and Iceland, became prevalent there after World War II. During the war, British troops occupied the Faroes, bringing with them the first dogs on the island. A Canadian survey of veterinarians, however, turned up no evidence of an association. The measles virus bears a resemblance to the distemper virus, and some scientists have suggested that what seems like measles antibodies in patients could in reality be distemper antibodies. Distemper has been known to infect humans but causes no visible disease. Recently a report in the *Scottish Medical Journal* once again suggested the link, reporting on four people with MS who as children had lived near each other in the same tenement block. One of the families was given a puppy that died of distemper. The playmates, of course, could also have shared a childhood disease. Despite all the suspicions that some virus is to blame for MS, no irrefutable proof of such a connection has been forthcoming yet.

As the search for the cause of MS goes on, doctors are already testing new approaches to treatment with drugs that act on the immune system. In 1983, at Harvard Medical School in Boston, neurologist Dr. Howard Weiner and his colleagues first showed that an immune-suppressant drug could halt progression of MS for at least a year. The drug, cyclophosphamide, long used as a cancer drug, worked in two-thirds of the MS patients. It damps down all cells of the immune system. The fact that it worked, even reversing disease effects in some, added to the evidence that MS is an auto-immune disease.

Following on Dr. Weiner's findings, a large trial of cyclophosphamide was begun in 20 medical centers in the U.S. and Canada, but will not be completed until 1990. It will take five years to determine if the drug has true lasting benefits for MS patients, because it can take years for the disease to progress. In Canada, a nation-wide study has begun in which treatment with cyclophosphamide is combined with plasma exchange (plasmapheresis), a procedure by which the liquid part of blood containing antibodies, but not the blood cells, is replaced. It involves 200 patients and will take three years.

Although cyclophosphamide is the first drug that has shown exciting success against MS, nobody considers it a total cure. The drug has toxic side-effects and doctors are reluctant to use it in young people, especially in early stages of MS. Within a year or two after treatment, MS begins progressing again and the patients need second or third courses of the therapy, adding to the worry about nasty effects from the drug over the long run.

Furthermore, not all cells of the immune system are involved in MS. "It's believed T cells sit at the heart of the disease," Dr. Weiner says. He is investigating treatment of patients with antibodies created in the laboratory, against T cells. The first such antibodies used were designed to take out of action all kinds of T cells. B cells are left untouched. The antibody was made against a particle (antigen) found on all varieties of Ts. When that gave encouraging results in the first group of patients, the scientists narrowed the range even more. They began trying antibodies that are specific only to T helper cells, leaving alone T suppressor cells that may be able to help stop an internal war on myelin. The hope is that specialized antibodies will be less toxic than immune-suppressant drugs and could safely be given to young patients before MS disables them.

In other experimental treatments, a different drug, called cyclosporine, is showing possibilities. Primarily used to prevent rejection of transplanted organs, it was the first drug devised that affected only T helper cells. Earlier immune-suppressant drugs knocked out the whole immune system. It is being tried in a cooperative study by 12 American medical centers. In mice, the drug reversed symptoms of a disease that is similar to MS and is used as a model to study the disease. The mouse counterpart of MS is called experimental auto-immune encephalomyelitis. In the study, about 40 patients at each center are given doses of the drug half as large as those used for transplant patients. Cyclosporine can cause side-effects, including kidney damage, when given in large doses. The patients are being closely monitored. Because patients can differ in their subjective description of symptoms, the effects on the disease are measured by means of a disability rating scale developed by the International Federation of Multiple Sclerosis Societies. Other studies with the drug are under way in Canada, West Germany, England, Denmark, and the Netherlands.

Interferon is another substance being tested in more than a dozen medical centers around the world as treatment for MS. It is produced in minuscule amounts naturally in the body. When a cell is infected with a virus, it secretes this protein, which helps stop the virus from reproducing itself. Interferon also increases the effectiveness of natural killer cells, macrophages, and cytotoxic T cells. If MS is the result of a persistent virus infection, interferon might be useful.

There are three known kinds of interferon: alpha, produced by all sorts of white cells (leukocytes); beta, produced by cells called fiberblasts; and gamma, produced by T and B cells only after they have recognized a virus and been turned on. When interferon was first discovered it was enormously expensive, because it had to be obtained from human cells where it is made in extremely tiny amounts. Now scientists have learned how to produce it in the laboratory by means of genetic engineering and it is more readily available. Different kinds of interferon are being tried against MS by various study groups, who are also testing different ways of injecting it. Early results of the effect on MS have not given a clear answer. The National Multiple Sclerosis Society in New York has said alpha interferon looks promising for some patients whose disease is remitting and relapsing, but not for those whose disease is steadily worsening.

A three-center study in California involving 24 patients who gave themselves daily injections of interferon for six months found 15 experienced fewer and milder attacks when compared with a six-month period in which they injected a fake interferon (placebo). All of the patients injected interferon during one phase of the study and placebo during another stage, but neither the patients nor their doctors knew who was getting which in each phase. The method is called a double blind study. At the beginning, keeping the patient from knowing whether or not the drug was real seemed unlikely. Interferon produces side-effects. Patients suffered fever, hair loss, fatigue, joint pain, loss of appetite, and depression — but mystifyingly, so did some of the patients being given the placebo. It's a phenomenon often seen with placebos in MS studies, doctors say. However, at the end of the two-year study, the 15 who had fewer attacks showed no improvement in overall effects on their nervous systems.

A study in British Columbia also showed encouraging preliminary results. When patients were given interferon, activity of cells that remove antibodies once they have done their job increased. Antibodies, although not the prime cause of myelin destruction, are typically found in high levels in the spinal fluid of MS patients and may contribute to the damage. It is not yet fully understood how interferon curbs flare-ups of the disease.

Yet another substance, still controversial, being tried in New York, is called copolymer I. Made by an immunologist at Weizmann Institute of Science in Israel, it is similar to myelin-basic protein and, at least in theory, is recognized by suppressor T cells, making them active so that they call a halt to the tissue damage being done by other immune cells. Several Canadian MS research clinics are gearing up to conduct studies of the substance in patients.

Overall, only one thing seems certain: the next five years will be peppered with discoveries about the nature of this baffling disease. There is justifiable hope for an end to the suffering it has been causing over many years and for an end to the frustrations of scientists it has stymied.

ARTHRITIS

In Canada alone, almost four million people have some form of arthritis. It has been making mankind ache for two million years, causing knees, hips, fingers, or other joints to be as hot, inflamed, and painful as if they'd been held to a searing fire. The most common form of the disease — of the more than 100 that come under the umbrella title of arthritis — is rheumatoid arthritis. For about 10 years, doctors have realized that it is an auto-immune disease; the damage being done to the body is the result of an attack by the very cells designed to protect it. In people with arthritis, B cells produce antibodies that attack perfectly healthy tissue. Surprisingly, we can all make these anti-self antibodies. The puzzle was why they only do damage to the tissue of joints in *some* people.

Recently, however, a new clue has been discovered that may explain why people with arthritis suffer damage while luckier people do not. At the University of Western Ontario in London, scientists found that healthy people have, in the bone marrow where B cells originate, a kind of cell that carries a molecule that blocks production of self-antibodies. In people with rheumatoid arthritis, these special cells with their important molecule are absent. That may allow abnormally high levels of so-called auto-antibodies to roam the body.

Why would we have auto-antibodies at all? Scientists

think we may need some of them to stick on worn out cells, earmarking them for removal by macrophages, our garbage collectors. Macrophages wouldn't eat old, damaged cells unless they were tagged with antibody. Researchers have found, for example, that aging red blood cells have sticking out from their outer coats an antigen for which we have auto-antibodies in the blood. This antigen is like a sign that says "Eat me." But too many auto-antibodies may spell trouble.

Antibodies, the Y-shaped weapons produced by B cells, can float in the circulation system for years, each keeping an eye open for the specific antigen that is the one shape the antibody matches. When an antigen is discovered and more antibodies are needed, T helper cells give the command for B cells to make them. When the danger is past, T suppressor cells stop production so antibodies won't clog up the blood-stream. At the University of Toronto, Dr. Catherine Lau, Dr. Edward Keystone, and colleagues have found that in people with arthritis, T suppressor cells were less able to release a chemical signal that says "Stop." In people with arthritis, auto-antibodies are formed against other antibodies circu-lating in their blood. Doctors call auto-antibodies that are attached to other antibodies "rheumatoid factor."

In healthy people if too many auto-antibodies were around, T suppressor cells would shut off the supply. But they don't do so in people with arthritis. There may not be enough T suppressor cells on hand to do the trick. Ordin-arily we have many more T helper cells available than suppressor cells. That's important, because if the immune system doesn't speed to the attack, a virus might get to the brain within seconds. Suppressor cells are produced in greater quantity when all alien signs (antigens) are gone, removed by antibodies. One possible new therapy for arthritis would be to make suppressor cells more effective or boost their numbers. Scientists are looking for ways to do just that.

One method may use chemicals that the immune cells produce to talk to each other, such as the stop signal, called suppressor-activating factor, and interleukin-2. Some evidence suggests arthritis patients produce a substance that interferes with interleukin-2, which is a crucial ingredient in the reproduction of T cells, including suppressor T cells.

Interferon is another part of the chemical language. In West Germany, almost by chance, doctors observed that injections of interferon seemed to relieve pain and swelling of rheumatoid arthritis in 28 of 38 patients. Now the clue is being investigated in other centers.

If you could look into the inflamed joint of an arthritis patient you'd see swarms of all kinds of immune cells and huge amounts of antibody being produced. Ordinarily, synovium, the joint tissue, is not a site where B cells produce antibodies. As well as destruction of synovium, widespread damage is being done to everything in sight, connective tissue and bone included. Swelling and pain result from the injury to the joint. Another innovative approach to treatment is concerned with reducing levels of substances produced by the body in response to injury. Within seconds of an injury, cells produce these materials that cause swelling and inflammation at the site. Among the substances are leukotrienes, made by white cells from a fatty acid. In San Francisco, Dr. Edward Goetzl recently discovered abnormally high levels of leukotrienes in patients with rheumatoid arthritis and in other types of arthritis such as gout and arthritic conditions of the spine. Leukotriene injected into a person causes pain. Now researchers are looking for a drug to block production of leukotriene, which in effect would be a new kind of pain killer for arthritics.

It has long been suspected there must be some connection between the nervous system and arthritis. The link may be a brain chemical scientists have dubbed "substance P." In 1984, a cooperative study by scientists in California and Massachusetts discovered substance P in high concentration in arthritic joints. They found if they injected the substance into arthritic rats, they could increase the severity of the disease. And they also found that substance P could directly stimulate B and T cells. Both Bs and Ts use substance P as a navigational aid, directing them to specific sites where they are needed. It's possible that by reducing the amount of substance P in arthritic joints, fewer immune cells would be attracted there, which would decrease the damage done by them.

As in other auto-immune diseases, a disease-causing organism has long been suspected of being the trigger in arthritis that sets off the self-attack. All sorts of viruses, such as the German measles virus, hepatitis B virus, and an array of common respiratory and digestive tract viruses, as well as some bacteria, have been identified as setting off some forms of arthritis. For example, doctors often see temporary inflammation in the joints of people suffering flu, mumps, or rubella (German measles). About 30 per cent of adult women given rubella vaccine have some joint reaction a week or so later. Such reactions are rarely seen in children after vaccination; however, some children who get rubella from playmates do have joint inflammation that sometimes recurs for months or even years. Scientists at the University of British Columbia have detected rubella virus still hiding in the joints months after the initial infection. They were also able to find the virus in the blood or synovial fluid of more than one-third of children with juvenile rheumatoid arthritis, suggesting a chronic rubella infection. The Canadian team also noted that animal studies have shown that certain cartilage cells may be where rubella viruses hide out. The virus can reproduce in them without killing the cells.

Bacteria are also known to infect joints, causing swelling and tenderness. The most common kind of bacteria that affects knees or other sites is the gonococcal bacteria that causes gonorrhea, but there are several others as well. With prompt treatment, soon after the first symptoms, bacterial arthritis can be cured without permanent damage to joints in the majority of cases.

Yet another indication that some germ is linked to rheumatoid arthritis came out of some medical detective work by Yale University doctors Allen Steere and Stephen Malawista. For seven years they tracked down the cause of Lyme disease, so called because the trail began in Old Lyme, Connecticut, where a cluster of children developed a rheumatic illness first thought to be juvenile rheumatoid arthritis. The children had something that looked like an insect bite, a clue that led to the discovery that a bacterium, carried by deer ticks, was the culprit in starting up the arthritis-like condition. Similarly, Australian scientists have found that a virus carried by a mosquito infects many people in the South Pacific, causing arthritis-like symptoms. Other organisms called mycoplasmas, tiny bacteria that can hide in synovial tissue, are also suspect and under intense investigation. Some researchers think bacteria may leave bits of themselves imbedded in cell walls, which keep acting as alarm signals to the immune system, even though the bacteria are dead. Unaware that what they discover are not living enemies, the immune cells keep up a persistent battle.

Another hot suspect is the Epstein-Barr virus, which causes mononucleosis. It is so common that nine in ten of us have encountered it at some time in our lives, although we may only have felt a bit tired and out of sorts as a result. California researchers have shown that people with rheumatoid arthritis have an abnormal response to the virus that blocks normal production of interferon. While almost everybody carries some lymphocytes infected with the E-B virus, arthritis patients have been found to have five times the average number of infected white cells, and some of them have E-B virus-infected cells in the synovial tissue. The E-B virus is known to stimulate the production of antibodies to other antigens as well as to its own and it may stimulate production of auto-antibodies. At the University of Toronto, however, studies indicate that the E-B virus may not cause arthritis. Mixing immune cells of patients with the virus in laboratory dishes, researchers discovered that the virus can show them cells that are already defective, although it did not cause the defect initially.

Yet another suspect is a small virus derived from a patient with severe arthritis in New York. Called RA-1, it was found to cause a rheumatoid-like illness in mice. Tests in the laboratory indicated that 13 of 14 arthritis patients had evidence of RA-1 in cells taken from synovial tissue. Scientists are now trying to learn more about this new virus.

Tracking down the guilty germ that triggers arthritis is important because, if there is one — or perhaps several different ones — a vaccine might be made. So far, the only treatment is to ease pain and inflammation. Says one Australian scientist, "We've been looking at the injuries caused by the far-flung shrapnel of rheumatoid arthritis. Now we're trying to find the fuse."

There are so many different kinds of arthritic conditions, it's probable that a number of germs are the culprits. Arthritis can follow infections of the urinary tract or the intestinal tract, usually showing up about a month later.

Some of the disease organisms are transmitted by sexual activity. Often the arthritis occurs in one knee. This kind of arthritis is sometimes called Reiter's syndrome, although doctors more often call it reactive arthritis. When doctors take white cells from the synovial fluid of such patients they find, by testing the cells in the laboratory, that they react most strongly with the germ that caused the infection. If doctors don't know which bug was the cause of the infection, testing the patient's white cells against a wide variety of germs may provide the answer. Such studies have given a clearer picture of reactive arthritis, implicating a number of infectious agents.

LUPUS

Lupus, or more formally, systemic lupus erythematosis, is another disease of the rheumatoid family that is almost certainly set off by an infection. So far, however, nobody knows which virus or bacterium it is. Immune cells go after connective tissue between organs, causing disorders that may include skin eruptions, arthritis, inflammation of the kidney and heart, which may affect other parts of the body, with the symptoms coming and going. It is most common in women aged 20 to 30. The female hormone estrogen appears to aggravate the disease, and women with lupus are wise to be wary of birth control pills. The trademark of lupus, although it is not seen in all patients, is a butterfly-shaped rash on the face.

While B cells of patients with lupus appear to have gone wild, relentlessly producing all sorts of antibodies, scientists think the underlying problem is that T helper cells have somehow gone wrong, a belief bolstered by the fact that in a similar disease in mice, antibodies against T helper cells injected into the mice stopped the disease from progressing. Such treatment would only be used in severe cases, because when T helper cells are knocked out of commission, the patient is more vulnerable to infections until the immune system rebuilds a supply of those cells.

Doctors at a number of medical centers are treating some lupus patients with radiation therapy, ordinarily thought of as treatment only for cancer. The radiation, emitted by a machine called a linear accelerator, is directed at parts of the body where white cells accumulate, such as lymph nodes and the spleen. In patients whose disease was damaging their kidneys and could have become life-threatening, the radiation stopped the damage and the patients have remained better, so far for four or more years. Damage to organs, such as kidneys, occurs because auto-antibodies, attaching themselves to other antibodies or white cells in the blood, are carried into small vessels in the kidneys, causing a traffic jam and creating havoc.

The goal scientists are seeking is a way to turn off, temporarily, the signal from T helper cells that is spurring continuous antibody production, without disrupting the whole normal immune response. But many things about the immune system remain mysterious, including the observation that rheumatoid arthritis is virtually never seen in people with Down's syndrome (once called Mongolism). Such people virtually never get multiple sclerosis, either, but they are more prone to diabetes, which is now also believed to be an auto-immune disease.

DIABETES

After heart disease and cancer, diabetes is the third biggest killer disease in North America. About one in 10 people with diabetes has the kind that must be controlled by injections of insulin and is called juvenile diabetes or, more commonly today, type I. It is the diabetes that children and young people typically develop. Until insulin was discovered in Toronto in 1921 by the late Sir Frederick Banting and Dr. Charles Best, there was little hope for patients who could not produce insulin in their bodies to control blood sugar levels. Insulin is produced in certain cells called Beta cells or islet cells in parts of the pancreas called Islets of Langerham. Without insulin, sugar can't get from the blood to cells that need sugar for fuel.

In the past few years doctors have learned that in patients with type I diabetes, something — possibly a virus — has tricked cells of the immune system into launching an attack on the Beta cells. In light of this surprising discovery, it may be possible within a few years, some doctors say, to prevent type I diabetes by stopping immune cells from destroying Beta cells.

Some preliminary studies have demonstrated that if patients are treated with a drug that halts rejection of transplanted organs as soon as the first symptoms of diabetes appear, it can protect the islet cells. At the University of Western Ontario, more than half of the first 30 patients treated with the drug cyclosporine, no longer needed insulin after a few weeks. Doctors can test blood serum for a piece of insulin called C-peptide to find out if Beta cells are working. Usually levels of the peptide decrease about three months after the onset of diabetes, indicating loss of insulin production. All patients in the study showed an increase in C-peptide, and physicians were able to reduce the amount of insulin injected in accordance with the peptide increase. Since then, a large study has been launched at seven Canadian and five European medical centers, involving 200 patients, to find out if those promising early findings hold up. The difficulty is that when the London patients were taken off the drug at the end of a year, their diabetes returned. If this treatment is to be successful, patients will have to take the drug for life. Like all powerful drugs, cyclosporine can have some bad effects and doctors are concerned about giving it to young people for long periods of time.

In London and Boston, doctors have begun treating small groups of people even before they show symptoms of diabetes but who are known to be at high risk (for instance if a brother or sister has diabetes). Two or more children in a family may have inherited the same pattern of immune-response genes that makes them sitting ducks for diabetes. A second high-risk factor is having antibodies to islet cells and sometimes also to insulin. The antibodies themselves don't cause diabetes but they indicate that the person is primed for the disease and that at some point, without treatment, the T cells that attack islet cells will become active. The third risk factor is evidence that a lower than average amount of insulin is being secreted. In New York, a seven-year study of 178 families in which one child already had diabetes found that these three distinct markers revealed which of 351 brothers and sisters of the patients were also likely to develop diabetes. Ten did; of these, all had two of the markers and eight had all three. Doctors estimate the likelihood of developing diabetes is 30 to 60 times greater for siblings of people with diabetes than for the general population. The genes they share contain the instructions that govern the way T cells and B cells will respond to a particular antigen. In a scientific study at the Joslin Diabetes Clinic in Boston, blood tests are offered free of charge to immediate family members of people with diabetes to determine if the relatives will likely develop the disease too. The aim is to compile a list of people at high risk who would get priority for any new method discovered to prevent diabetes from developing.

It's probable that people prone to diabetes make a response to something on or inside the islet cell that immune cells have mistakenly identified as foreign because it looks like a virus antigen. At the University of Calgary, doctors have identified a virus they believe causes diabetes in some of the people who have inherited vulnerability to the disease. It is a coxsackie virus — one of a group of viruses first identified in Coxsackie, N.Y. The virus causes influenza-like symptoms. The Alberta doctors found it had caused inflammation of the pancreas in 20 per cent of a group of children, ages four to 14, who developed diabetes. Some doctors say the trigger could have been pulled long before symptoms of the disease appear. Some people are known to have antibodies to their own islet cells for many years without obvious disease. Diabetes is often first diagnosed in a child following an infectious disease, flu, or some other stressful illness, but destruction of the Beta cells may have begun occurring silently much earlier.

For people who have diabetes, there is high hope that transplanting islet cells will restore the source of insulin. Attempts to transplant the pancreas have been moderately successful, but patients only need Beta cells replaced; some patients have been given just those cells with promising outcomes. A major difficulty researchers faced was obtaining pure islet cells from the pancreas. Scientists even took pancreatic tissue on a space flight, hoping the cells might be easier to pry loose from the tissue in zero gravity.

At Washington University in St. Louis, Missouri, Dr. Paul Lacey dug out of his attic an old hand-cranked meat grinder and used it to mince pancreas before he filtered out islet cells. He tried a Cuisinart, but it didn't work, he confided later to reporters. The human pancreas contains many thousands of islet cells. Putting a supply of these tiny cells, each about a millimeter in size, into a diabetic does not require major surgery. They are not even put into the pancreas because they can produce insulin as well in other locations and are thought to be safer elsewhere. Doctors are trying different locations, such as the portal vein leading to the liver, and between membranes that attach the bowel to the body. At one medical center they are implanted in the spleen, despite the fact that the spleen is a gathering spot for immune cells — it seems rather like putting a chicken into a den of foxes! A trial of such transplants is progressing in four U.S. medical centers.

Transplanted islet cells, however, may need to be hidden from the immune system, or suffer the fate of the originals. In Toronto, islet cells have been tucked into tiny capsules where they are protected from attack by the patient's immune system. Studies in animals have shown that a single injection of such capsules can provide insulin as it is needed for at least a year; the technique may be ready to test in people in the near future.

THYROID DISEASE

Graves' disease, marked by an overactive thyroid gland and sometimes by bulging eyes, and Hashimoto's thyroiditis, an underactivity of the thyroid, are relatively common auto-immune diseases. Graves' disease is far more common in women than in men, usually occurring between the ages of 20 and 40. Hashimoto's thyroiditis, once thought to be very rare, is now known to affect three or four of every 100 people and many others, particularly older women, may have it without showing outward symptoms.

Some doctors think Hashimoto's thyroiditis has become more frequent in the past few decades because of the increase in iodine in the typical North American diet, which contains two to five times as much iodine as recommended by dieticians. Recent experiments have shown that iodine fed to certain strains of chickens that are prone to thyroiditis will bring on the disease. Hashimoto's thyroiditis was one of the first auto-immune diseases recognized, and was investigated more than 30 years ago when scientists in England found high levels of antibodies to thyroid tissue in the blood of patients.

Since then, different kinds of auto-antibodies have been found in patients with these diseases. One kind in particular interested researchers and it turned out to be a landmark discovery in the puzzle of auto-immunity. This type of antibody makes thyroid cells behave as if they had been given a hormone that stimulates thyroid activity. The hormone is the body's natural way of telling the thyroid gland to get busy. Thyroid cells have receptors on their surfaces that await the hormone message. But researchers found that in thyroid patients auto-antibodies attached themselves to the receptors, making the thyroid cell respond as it would to the hormone signal. The result was chronic stimulation of the gland, causing it to be overly active. These auto-antibodies have been found in almost all patients with Graves' disease. The thyroid gland plays an important role in growth of children and in body metabolism, but a person with Graves' disease may seem as if her motor is running too fast, causing weight loss, restlessness, weakness, and tremors.

Conversely, other auto-antibodies, although they also latch onto the thyroid cells' hormone receptors, don't stimulate the gland. Indeed they do the opposite: they simply block out the thyroid-stimulating message. Hormone can't get to the receptors because antibodies are in the way. The result may be an under-active thyroid. Yet another auto-antibody promotes abnormal growth of the gland and may explain goiter, a swelling in the neck that can occur in patients with either under- or over-active thyroids.

Why are these auto-antibodies produced? That is not yet known, but scientists have discovered a substance in a bacterium that is like the receptor. The bacterium is called Yersinia enterocolitica, an impressive name for a rather ordinary intestinal tract germ. People with Graves' disease often have evidence in their blood of infection by this bacterium. Another possible clue is the recent finding at the University of Chicago that a protein produced in the thyroid may be an antigen that starts off the production of auto-antibodies. The protein is an enzyme called peroxidase. It's possible that most people can produce antibodies against this enzyme but production is kept under tight rein by T suppressor cells. But patients with Graves' disease typically have reduced numbers of suppressor cells. (As they get better and their thyroid glands return to normal, levels of suppressor cells are also found to be increasing.)

Scientists have found that in both kinds of thyroid disease patients appear to have some defect regulating the supply of T suppressor cells. Doctors sometimes see spontaneous recoveries of people with Graves' disease and believe that these people have had their immune systems temporarily knocked out of kilter by an infection or stress. When the stress or infection is over, defense mechanisms return to normal and the thyroid problem disappears.

It seems highly probable that the genes governing the immune system also play a role in thyroid disease. Like other auto-immune diseases, they often run in families and in identical twins (whose genes are the same). If one of the twins has thyroid disease, in a high percentage of cases the other will also have it. But it doesn't happen in 100 per cent of these cases, so doctors know there is some other factor triggering the disease as well as the genes.

Scientists have found that about half of the people with auto-immune thyroid disease have a pattern of immune system genes that may be linked to particular susceptibility. But as yet the picture is not really clear. Some studies show that families with particular gene patterns have a number of members with auto-immune diseases, but different members may have different forms of disease or more than one kind. Even the bulging eyes that often accompany Graves' disease may well be caused by a separate disease. Auto-antibodies to particles of eye muscle have been found in Graves' patients whose eyes are affected, but not in those without protruding eyes, a symptom previously believed to be part and parcel of Graves' disease.

Women who are susceptible to thyroid diseases frequently have a flare-up of the condition following pregnancy. Swedish scientists have reported thyroid disease after pregnancy in about six per cent of women. It is believed that because during pregnancy a woman's immune response is kept damped down so it won't attack the baby whose cells might be seen as foreign, there may be a rebound afterwards as immune cells return to a more vigorous state. At that time the supply of antibodies, including thyroid auto-antibodies, may increase to the point where the thyroid is affected. The condition is usually temporary.

MYASTHENIA GRAVIS

Like Graves' disease, myasthenia gravis is a condition in which auto-antibodies, and possibly T cells, interfere with and destroy receptors on certain cells. In this rare disease, however, it is receptors on muscle fibers that come under attack. When you want a muscle to contract, nerves release a substance called acetylcholine, which is normally received by receptors on the outer covering of muscle fibers. But people with myasthenia have only 20 per cent or so of the normal number of receptors. Doctors can find evidence that immune cells have attacked the receptors. They also find decreased numbers of T suppressor cells, which ordinarily would stop such attacks. Furthermore, doctors believe that the thymus is involved in some way not yet understood. But about 10 per cent of such patients have a growth on the thymus gland, and it has also been found that removing the thymus, whether or not there is a growth there, relieves the condition in most patients with severe disease affecting all parts of their bodies.

However, auto-antibodies seem to be the main culprits, causing the muscle weakness and fatigue that mark this disease. Being given blood serum from a patient with myasthenia could cause the condition. Babies born to women with myasthenia sometimes have it temporarily after birth while they still have antibodies from their mothers. Oddly, the disease affects young women and elderly men most often, although it is only seen in a handful of people among each million in the population. Sometimes patients are treated with plasmapheresis, which gets rid of the unwanted antibodies circulating in the blood by exchanging the patient's blood plasma with substitute plasma. In other cases, immune-suppressant drugs, such as cyclosporine, steroids, asathioprine, or cyclophosphamide, are used. Recent reports say that cyclosporine has shown impressive results.

BLOOD DISORDERS

Aplastic anemia, a life-threatening condition in which the bone marrow is unable to produce a sufficient supply of red blood cells, is, at least in some cases, almost certainly an auto-immune disease. However, there is evidence that patients with this condition, rather than having too few T suppressor cells, as is the case in a number of auto-immune conditions, have too many T suppressor cells acting on the bone marrow to prevent red cell formation. Ordinarily, red cells are produced and die with incredible speed. A healthy person produces about three million red cells per second and about the same number die in that brief time. Researchers have found that different subgroups of T cells play a part in keeping the red cell balance — some of them encouraging the production of red cells, some of them slowing production down. Now there is evidence that in the bone marrow of these patients where all blood cells, red and white, originate, the balance has been lost because T suppressor cells and natural killer cells have become too numerous or too strong. Recently, scientists at the U.S. National Institutes of Health have discovered that interferon, secreted by cells infected with a virus, may be implicated in causing aplastic anemia. This indicates that the disease might begin with a virus infection. Interferon slows cell proliferation down and also may turn on both T suppressor cells and natural killer cells.

It isn't yet known how many patients with aplastic anemia have disease caused in this way. But about 40 per cent of them improve when treated with immune-suppressant drugs, such as cyclophosphamide or steroids. Doctors originally saw the benefit when such patients were given immune-suppressants prior to having a bone marrow transplant. Such transplants may give patients a brand new healthy blood-forming system.

Other kinds of anemias, such as pernicious anemia and haemolytic anemia, are also auto-immune diseases. With pernicious anemia, patients make self-antibodies against an enzyme called intrinsic factor, which is essential in the production of normal red blood cells. Haemolytic anemia may result when auto-antibodies are formed against red cells themselves.

Another blood problem, called thrombocytopenic purpura, involves bleeding due to a decrease in the number of platelets in the blood and may show up as bruises or purple patches under the skin. It is caused by antibodies that are produced against platelet antigens. Platelets, small disc-shaped particles in the blood, are vital to blood clotting. But in this condition, platelets covered with such antibodies are quickly cleared out of the bloodstream. In the last little while, doctors have been seeing this problem in homosexual men, some of them with AIDS. Previously, the condition was seen primarily in girls and women.

Since 1981, physicians have known that this platelet disease can be treated successfully by giving patients intravenous transfusions of immunoglobulin (antibodies), a preparation made from blood plasma obtained from thousands of healthy blood donors. No one knows for sure why it works, but researchers suggest that present in the donors' blood are antibodies fitting the patient's auto-antibodies. These antibodies prevent the problem by blocking the auto-antibodies from attaching themselves to the platelet antigens. It may be that in all healthy people auto-antibodies are partly kept in check by means of other antibodies.

Immunoglobulin preparations have also been tested against other auto-immune diseases with some success. For example, some patients with the bleeding disease, hemophilia, lack the clotting substance called Factor VIII because their systems make auto-antibodies against it. In these patients the levels of the trouble-makers dropped rapidly after immunoglobulin transfusion.

EYE DISEASES

Doctors call inflammation of the inner portions of the eye, uveitis. In North America it has been estimated to be the cause of 10 per cent of serious vision loss. In a relatively small number of cases, an infectious organism can be identified as the cause, but what causes the inflammation in the first place is often unknown. Bleeding and swelling in the eye can result in deterioration of sight. Ordinarily, immune cells leave the eye alone. They seem to be keenly aware that eye tissue is self and to be treated with kid gloves.

But scientists have found that the retina, which receives the image of objects you see, contains particles that can bring a reaction from T cells in some people. The finding has led to trials of treatment with the drug cyclosporine, which halts helper T cell activity, with encouraging early results. Recently researchers have also found a second protein, identical to the retina-antigen, in rods of the eye. Rods, nerve cells in the retina, are largely responsible for black and white vision. (Their partner cells, called cones, look after color vision.)

OTHER AILMENTS

Some 50 diseases, once of unknown origin, are today included on the list of ailments considered auto-immune diseases. Some men may be unable to father children because their sperm comes under attack by the immune system. Skin diseases, such as the rare blistering condition called epidermolysis bullosa, may result from auto-antibodies being formed to proteins in the underlying layers of skin. Some doctors consider psoriasis a condition in which T cells get a message wrong from dendritic cells in the skin, cells which, like macrophages, present antigens to the T cells to be identified.

Possibly the most recent addition to the list is narcolepsy, a disease marked by sudden, uncontrollable urges to sleep many times a day. Until 1985 everyone had presumed it was a kind of nerve disorder, though no defects were found in the brain. Then researchers in England, Canada, France, Japan, and the U.S. looked at the immune response genes of patients. They found that among 150 patients, all but two had one particular gene that is ordinarily found in only one person in five in the general population. The finding indicated that narcolepsy could well be an auto-immune disease, and extensive investigation of the immune systems of patients is being conducted at a number of research centers. In Montreal, scientists have focused on brain chemicals that transmit messages, called dopamine and serotonin, suspecting there may be something about them that could provide an explanation. Both have an effect on immune cells.

Gout, like other arthritis diseases, results from an

attack on self-tissue. But some scientists think the problem here is the shape of the particle that macrophages try to engulf. Patients with gout produce uric acid crystals, sharp, needle-like structures. Macrophages have little trouble taking in round shapes, such as bacteria, but sharp shapes may be a different matter. Some researchers in Britain say that the chemicals that macrophages use to break down an "enemy" they've scooped up may leak out into surrounding tissue when the macrophage can't engulf its prey completely. These chemicals, which the macrophage fires, then hit the wrong targets, parts of the body the macrophage is trying to protect. The chemicals may do damage to joints. Immune cells are directed to damaged tissue and the ensuing battle is gout.

Considering the short period of time in which scientists have had techniques that let them examine in detail genes, molecules, chemicals, and activities of the cells of the immune system, it is astounding how many discoveries have been made. But as almost every researcher will tell you, they've also learned what a vast amount remains shrouded in fog. Yet already the possibilities for totally new forms of treatment can be seen. Few today would consider it madness to predict, within our lifetimes, that we'll see the disappearance of an array of diseases presently afflicting millions of people and diminishing their enjoyment of life by the pain and disabilities they cause.

CHAPTER 4

Stress: The Brain-Immune System Connection

In 1979, three years after the accident at Three Mile Island nuclear plant, a psychologist who had been studying residents of the area noted that many of them were still suffering high levels of stress and also a lot of illnesses. But their doctors reported that the illnesses were not the effects of radiation; the people were sick with infections of the respiratory tract. Studies of the immune systems of more than 30 of them disclosed low levels of T cells and B cells.

The findings added one more bit of evidence to an increasing number of studies that have demonstrated a link between stress and body defenses. You may have noticed that you or others in your family seem most susceptible to colds when under considerable pressure. For many years, patients and doctors have observed that diseases frequently follow grief, the misery of unrequited love, financial losses, severe humiliation, or other painful events. Some doctors say that one of the first questions they ask a sick patient in the process of diagnosis is, "What has been going on in your personal life?"

As long ago as 1937, Canada's famous stress expert, the late Dr. Hans Selye, reported that stress brought about a drop in the number of lymphocytes — later identified as T and B cells — in the blood. But for the most part, scientists did not think there was a connection between the brain and the immune system. Immune cells, it was believed, acted independently in response to the entry of germs or other antigens that managed to get into the body. After all, in a test tube, immune cells reacted to antigens and obviously no brain was on hand to tell them to do so. For years, doctors believed that this was evidence that the immune system and the nervous system were quite separate. More recently, studies in many medical centers have discovered that there are connections between the two. But at first the scientists didn't know whether the immune system cells were talking to the brain or were just listening for signals from the body's central command in the head. Today they have learned that there is communication back and forth between the two.

Certain cells of your immune system send chemical messages to the nervous system, providing information about the presence of an intruder and the site of the invasion. Your sensory mechanisms of touch, sight, hearing, and smell provide a steady flow of information to the brain about substances affecting the body, such as pressure sensations from the seat you are sitting on or the stickiness of the jam you got on your finger. Likewise, the immune system also relays information, telling the brain about things that sensory mechanisms can't detect. You couldn't feel, see, hear, or smell a cold virus land in your nose, but it won't be long before an immune cell knows it is there.

An infected cell sends out a cry of alarm in the form of interferon. That brings in the first battalions of troops. But researchers have discovered that nerve cells also have receptors for interferon and so can receive the warning message. Interferon was discovered to be like a hormone produced by the pituitary gland by Dr. Edwin Blalock of the University of

Alabama, Birmingham, and colleagues at the University of Texas, Galveston. The hormone, ACTH (adrenocorticotropic hormone), brings about release of steroids; the scientists found interferon can act the same way.

The brain has a direct line of communication to the spleen, lymph nodes, and other immune system organs. Nerve endings are located in all of them. The nervous system is like a telephone network ceaselessly carrying countless messages back and forth. When a message received by the brain says the body is in danger, clusters of cells in a part of the brain called the hypothalamus produce certain peptides, small protein molecules, which launch a cascade of hormones that are commonly called stress hormones. From the pituitary gland come hormones that cause the adrenal gland to pour out steroid hormones. Your heart races and you breathe harder. For the time being, other body functions, such as digestion, are postponed so that all energy can be directed toward escape or physical combat — the fight or flight reaction.

These corticosteroid hormones suppress the immune system. A discovery that surprised many scientists was that lymphocytes had on their surfaces receptors for the hormones, meaning that they could receive such messages. Like other systems that are given a temporary halt order, the immune system, too, gets the signal to wait. Nature presumably designed things that way. At the moment of danger, it is more important to get you away from the tiger's jaws than to worry about the bacteria on its teeth!

Doctors knew that the immune system is suppressed when a person suffers severe burns or injuries, causing physical stress. But only recently have they devised studies to determine if mental stress has an impact on the immune system similar to the effects of stress from physical damage. When a person is under acute stress today, the cause is not likely to be life-threatening physical danger, yet the mechanisms of response to stress remain the same. The immune system is put on hold. Logically, then, at a time of stress, a person may well be more vulnerable to invasion by a germ. But what proof can science uncover that this is so?

There's no doubt that steroids can put the brakes on the immune system, and stress hormones are steroids. Doctors make use of this ability of steroid hormones to damp down the immune system by using steroid drugs in the treatment of some auto-immune diseases, and to prevent rejection of transplanted organs. The drugs act on immune cells only because the cells have receptors for them.

It was a surprise to find that lymphocytes had receptors for hormones by which to receive messages from the brain. It was even more surprising to discover that these white cells could tell the brain things, too. Certain lymphocytes, after an infection is under control, secrete hormone-like substances themselves, apparently telegraphing the news of the victory. Swiss scientists have discovered that a distinct electrical pattern shows up in your brain when you are immunized. "The brain is informed of the immunization," says one of the discoverers, Dr. Hugo Besedovsky. In many ways, says another scientist, a lymphocyte is like a floating nerve cell. Indeed, there are many similarities between the immune system and the nervous system: both can learn from experience and remember, both can detect and respond to an infinite array of stimulations, and both make chemicals in order to communicate.

The brain doesn't restrict itself to hormones as its messengers. So far scientists have found some 60 brain chemicals that play this role and they say many more are still to be identified. Some of them, such as serotonin and dopamine, which are important in the brain, are known as neurotransmitters. Studies have now shown that these, too, have an impact on the immune system. If serotonin levels are elevated, for example, the immune response is suppressed. Dopamine, on the other hand, appears to stimulate the immune system. People with Parkinson's disease, sometimes called shaking palsy, have too little dopamine. Some studies found a deficiency in T cells in such patients. Research with mice found that if the part of the brain that produces compounds like dopamine was damaged, the stem cells in bone marrow, which are the forefathers of immune cells, declined.

Natural pain killers, similar to opiates such as morphine and tranquilizers such as Valium, are also produced in the brain. Astonishingly, lymphocytes have receptors for receiving these messages, too. Research has shown that intense stress, which cannot be escaped, can bring on production of the brain's built-in opiates (called endorphins). Scientists at the University of Colorado found that animals subjected to acute stress were less sensitive to pain because these natural opiates were produced. Studies at the University of Michigan have showed that the brain's own pain killers suppress the immune system. When scientists blocked the receptors on the lymphocytes, preventing the pain-killer message from getting through, there was no suppression of the immune cell activity.

Brain chemicals called peptides, are also messengers. One of them, called substance P, can be received by T helper cells. Researchers at the University of California in San Francisco discovered that substance P makes the immune system more active at particular sites in the body. Among those sites are joints in the body commonly affected in people with rheumatoid arthritis. Studying arthritic joints, the scientists found high concentrations of substance P. If they injected the substance into the arthritic leg joint of rats, the severity of the arthritis increased. Nature evidently intends substance P to help the immune cells get to the scene of an infection, because the substance opens up blood vessels, allowing lymphocytes to enter the area faster. But in an auto-immune disease like arthritis, it makes matters worse. Investigators are examining ways of slowing down production of substance P as a possible new treatment for arthritis, and also for asthma, a condition in which it may also play a part. But it will be some time yet before they understand the roles of the substance well enough to be sure such treatment wouldn't do harm elsewhere in the immune system. It may be a key signal from which lymphocytes locate an invasion of germs. Lymphocytes can swim against the flow of blood and wiggle through tissue in response to a call from any part of the body under siege.

University of Toronto studies have showed that another peptide, which is a neurotransmitter relaying signals in the intestines, calls lymphocytes to a trouble spot in that part of the digestive tract. This homing mechanism is called vaso-active intestinal peptide, or VIP, a short-form of its name that may be very appropriate: it is possibly a Very Important Peptide in body defenses.

The fact that a brain chemical can modify a person's mood and also act on immune cells may indicate a link between emotions and body defenses. Some studies have found that people suffering severe depression have significantly lower numbers of immune cells. But they don't find that true of people with schizophrenia. Researchers at the U.S. National Institute of Mental Health have also found receptors in immune cells for anti-anxiety substances produced by the brain. These, too, reduce immune cell activity. People who are depressed or extremely anxious may unwittingly be weakening their own body defenses, or perhaps throwing them out of balance.

Drugs used to treat mental disorders resemble the brain's natural chemicals. That's why they have an effect. In the course of evolution, nature did not have a crystal ball that said that one day humans would take drugs like morphine and tranquilizers. Thus it did not provide receptors for them. In fact, it is the other way around: the drugs work because they are just like natural products of the brain. But now doctors are realizing they must take into account the effects of such drugs on body defenses. For example, lithium, used to treat depression, has been found to influence the actions of suppressor T cells. These cells are like the brakes of the immune system. If they aren't working properly, an auto-immune disease in which ordinary body tissue is attacked may develop. For 20 years, it has been known that some people taking lithium develop thyroid disease, which doctors have established fairly solidly as an auto-immune disease. It doesn't seem to happen however, unless the person taking lithium is set up for the disease by already having in their system some antibodies against their own thyroid tissue. Then, if the brakes fail, the auto-antibodies roll into action.

Overall, it is becoming clear that the brain has many ways of making an impact on the immune system. Conversely, susbstances produced by lymphocytes, such as interferon and interleukin, can act on nerves, making nerve cells fire.

Undoubtedly, there is a lot of chatter, back and forth, between the central nervous system and the immune system. But the surface has only been skimmed so far in determining what effect the communication has on a person's health. Research continues on just what happens in the immune system when the brain perceives stress. A variety of animal experiments have shown quite clearly that stress can temporarily lower both T cells and B cells. Researchers have measured the effects on immune cells in mice exposed to stressful noise, light, and housing conditions, and in young monkeys separated from their mothers or from playmates. For a couple of weeks, immune responses were weaker. But the immune systems returned to normal as the mice grew accustomed to the noise or crowding, and as the monkeys were reunited with parent or friend.

Our emotions being so complex, it would scarcely be possible to measure in humans the exact connection between a given type of stress and the immune system. However, several studies of bereaved people after their spouses had died found immune responses reduced in the first two months. Most, but not all, of the grieving people showed a return to normal after that period, although it took up to a year for some. But some scientists questioned whether the cause might be the result of factors other than emotions, possibly changes in nutrition, sleep, and exercise that might weaken defenses. However, in one study of 15 men whose wives had died of breast cancer after lengthy illnesses, the men said they had not changed their own daily habits when their wives died. The men had accepted some time earlier the impending loss of their wives, and the death had not abruptly disrupted their lives or made them unable to eat or sleep. Yet they showed the same reduced immune responses as bereaved people in other studies who were less prepared for their loss.

Less severe stress has also been shown to affect body defenses. A study of dental students found that at the time of final examinations, IgA antibodies in their saliva fell. Since these are front-line defenders against respiratory illnesses, the students could have been more apt to get colds. The study also found that those students who were the most intense personalities — who were most worried about doing well on their exams — took longer to return to normal antibody levels. In other words, those under the most stress at exam time were the ones whose immune systems were upset the most. This squares with the reports of a Harvard University psychologist who devised a test to determine the kind of personality most affected by stress. He reported that his test showed the people hardest hit were those who had a great need for power but whose drive to obtain it was thwarted. Such people, he said, were more often stricken with respiratory infections as well as high blood pressure, a common condition in people under stress.

At Yale University in the late 1970s, West Point cadets were studied for their susceptibility to mononucleosis (sometimes called the kissing disease and common in colleges). Over a period of years, it was found that one-fifth of them developed antibodies to the virus each year, but that only one in four of those showed symptoms and felt sick. A comparison of the sick and non-sick cadets revealed that those who got sick tended to be ambitious, intensely wanting military careers but doing poorly in their academic work. The comparison suggested that those under the most stress were the ones who fell ill.

Still other investigators have discovered low levels of natural killer cells in lonely students and in some residents of nursing homes who felt abandoned by their families. Natural killer cells play a key part in ridding the body of cancer cells, as well as holding the fort for the first few days after an infection while the rest of the body's soldiers mobilize. In animal studies at the University of Colorado, natural killer cells removed from rats exposed to stress, when grown in culture dishes with tumor cells, were less effective in killing those cells than were natural killer cells from other rats. Women with breast cancer who had low levels of natural killer cells, according to another study, tended to be the ones who had little hope that they could be cured of their disease.

But we should not jump to conclusions. Much of the evidence linking stress and the immune system is circumstantial. Despite many studies showing that stress has an impact on the numbers or effectiveness of T cells and B cells, there is little solid proof that people whose immune cells are altered in some way will, inevitably, become ill. Some researchers have discovered that people with exceedingly low levels of different kinds of immune cells were perfectly healthy. Studies of astronauts revealed that though their immune cell levels were lower after the stress of splashdown on their return to earth, they didn't become ill.

One patient with AIDS, the fearful disease that knocks the stuffing out of the immune system, did not have so much as a cold in two and a half years after his disease was diagnosed. Maybe he was unbelievably lucky and never encountered a germ. Or maybe there is an explanation as yet completely hidden from science. Nevertheless, doctors may learn from AIDS patients a great deal about the interaction between emotions and body defenses. There is no question that these patients are under great stress, and they already have impaired immune systems. As one doctor said "They face a double challenge." Researchers have begun studies to determine if there is a measurable factor in AIDS patients who live five years that helps them cope emotionally with their situation and so protects them from infections. A New York psychiatrist has said that people with pre-AIDS, who don't know what the future will bring, are under even more stress than those whose diagnosis of AIDS has been confirmed. "They live with impending doom," she said. "They wait for the other shoe to drop." It is estimated that about 17 per cent of those with the pre-AIDS condition will go on to develop full-blown AIDS. So far, doctors can't say if from among this group those who suffer the most stress will be more likely to get AIDS, but they do hope to find out. Measures to counter stress, such as relaxation techniques or meditation, might then become a useful addition to therapy.

Your immune system also may play a part in putting you to sleep each night. In animals, interleukin-1, the substance produced by macrophages and certain other cells, promotes deep (slow-wave) sleep. To determine if that was also true in man, Dr. Harvey Moldofsky and colleagues at the University of Toronto investigated the immune cells in blood of volunteers over a 24-hour period, while they were awake and asleep. They found interleukin-1 activity increased at the onset of sleep; following that came an increase in interleukin-2, secreted by T cells. Natural killer cells, however, became less active during sleep. "These observed sleep-related immunologic activities might relate to the restorative function of sleep," says Dr. Moldofsky. Perhaps inability to sleep, often the plight of people under severe stress, contributes to the suppression of the immune system by stress. Shakespeare knew of the value of untroubled sleep: Lady Macbeth describes it as "innocent sleep, sleep that knits up the ravell'd sleeve of care . . . balm of hurt minds . . ." Sleep, soothing the mind, may also help the immune system protect the body.

Scientists have demonstrated the existence of a pathway that links a part of the brain, the hypothalamus (located between the two brain hemispheres), with the thymus gland, where T cells mature. When a person is under stress, the hypothalamus releases a chemical, inducing the pituitary to secrete a hormone that, in turn, orders the adrenal glands to release steroid hormones into the bloodstream. In small doses, steroid hormones spur the immune response. But in large doses, they damage or destroy immature T cells under development in the thymus gland. Or they cause the T cells to leave the thymus too soon, before they are ready to work effectively. The thymus, once bulging with T cells, shrinks dramatically. The thymus makes hormones, collectively called thymosin, discovered by Dr. Allan Goldstein and Dr. Nicholas Hall of George Washington University in Washington, D.C. Certain thymosins help young T cells become specialized T helper, T killer, or T suppressor cells. Recently the two doctors discovered that some thymosins act on the hypothalamus and the pituitary gland, helping regulate steroids and telling the brain what is going on in body defenses.

Is there anything we can do for ourselves to keep stress from diminishing our immune systems? We get a clue from animal studies. Researchers found that stress didn't reduce immune cells in rats, if the rats could control the stress. In one experiment, for example, rats could avoid the stress of a slight electric shock by turning a wheel in their cage. They quickly learned the trick of avoiding shocks much of the time, and their immune systems were not affected. Similar rats, who had no control over the shocks but were actually given no more than the first group, showed a drop in immune response. Some psychologists say that people who believe that they can control stressful circumstances, even if they really can't, seem to retain their usual immune defenses. "It is as if thoughts that run through the mind may also course through the body," one scientist has said.

People who feel helpless and unable to cope with stress are more likely to be depressed and anxious, and depression, as mentioned earlier, has been linked, fairly clearly, with a depressed immune system. In a small study, Dr. Nicholas Hall, co-discoverer of thymosin, found that cancer patients can increase their T cells by following a regime of "guided imagery" — visualizing their immune systems being turned on in the same way Olympic athletes prepare for competitions by thinking through every motion, enabling them to clear a hurdle by an extra half-inch. Dr. Hall says there is no proof that the increase in T cells has an impact on their cancers. "But these people feel good," he says. They become less depressed and withdrawn.

The patients select their own images. "Some are quite military, some pastoral." Dr. Hall adds that one patient, who could not bring himself to kill anything, even cancer cells that might kill him, imagined his body as a garden where he watered and nourished flowers (white cells) and ignored weeds (cancer cells). Monthly testing of the patients' blood, over an 18-month period, provided the first scientific proof that people can use thoughts to increase immune cells, possibly improving defenses against infections to which cancer patients are prone, even if their tumors are unchanged. And elated that they are not helpless pawns of their disease, such patients are lifted out of depression.

Recently, one of the first studies to connect depression, immune suppression, and a disease was completed at the University of California. It revealed that people who repeatedly had herpes frequently had a recurrence when they were depressed. Scientists monitoring the patients' blood could see, when patients first became depressed, levels of immune cells going down some time before the herpes sores developed. Many herpes patients say they suffer outbreaks of the sores when they are under stress. The California study didn't find that stress brought on the recurrences but suggests that the trigger was the person's attitude to the stressful event, not the event itself. If the stress left the person mired in melancholy, the herpes virus might gain the advantage.

Some people seem to be inherently better than others at coping with stress. Their pain may be as great, yet they are able to regain control of their emotional upheavals, while others go on being emotionally bruised and battered even after the acute period of stress is over. Do the lucky ones have brain cells that turn on production of mood-altering chemicals more rapidly? And does that, in turn, keep the immune system in proper balance? Nobody knows yet. But if the seemingly incredible finding of one University of California researcher is correct, we may all have some control over those brain chemicals. He found that facial expressions — smiles and frowns — can spark nerve cells in the brain and produce brain chemicals that alter moods. He suggests that the brain responds to the body signal, just as the face responds with a smile or frown to a happy or sad thought. It's possible that the brain relays the message to other parts of the body, even to the cells of the immune system. Whether it is proven true or not remains to be seen, but it's a lovely thought that a smile might help ward off a cold germ. Can it hurt to give it a try?

CHAPTER 5

Aging and Sex Differences in Immunity

How old you are and whether you are male or female makes a difference in how your body defenses work. Why? That has long been a mystery and much of the mystery remains today. Yet some parts of the picture are beginning to emerge, providing glimpses that make scientists and the rest of us impatient to learn more.

With aging comes an increased risk of cancer. And elderly people are more susceptible to infections that don't clear up when treated with drugs that are usually effective. Indeed, at one time, pneumonia was sometimes called the "old person's friend" because it brought an end to a prolonged and painful period of dying. For both those reasons — the increase in cancer and in infectious diseases —

doctors suspected that the immune system fails in old age. Yet, at the same time, old people are more likely to have arthritis, an auto-immune disease, indicating active, albeit misguided, B cells and T cells. And the longer people had lived, the more germs or other antigens one might expect they had encountered and would therefore be immune to. Little was known about the process of aging at all, much less about the effects of aging on immune cells. Only in recent years have scientists begun extensive investigation into what growing old is all about within the cells that make up the body. In fact, the special field of medicine called gerontology or geriatrics, the study of aging and medical care for the elderly, has only become recognized in the past few years. In the western world, more and more people are living to ripe old ages. At the turn of the century, the average lifespan was only 45 years. But at that time, many children and young people died of infectious diseases that medical science has since brought under control. A baby born today has a life expectancy of well over 70 years, and more people than ever before live into their 80s and 90s. Not surprisingly, with an ever-growing segment of the population becoming senior citizens, interest in aging blossomed.

In general, scientists believe the human body has a built-in limit to the length of time it can survive, and that limit is about 100 years, maybe at most 115. Few of us would complain if we could live that long in vigorous good health.

Some 20 years ago, American scientist Dr. Leonard Hayflick said normal cells seemed programmed such that they could divide to reproduce themselves only a given number of times. Doctors have found that in the aged, healthy cells in organs and tissues have been partly replaced by scar tissue. Cells have the capacity to renew themselves for about a century, because most cells of the body in an adult don't need to divide too often unless there is injury to the tissue they form. All cells in any given organ or tissue don't reach the end of their capacity at the same time because they are a mixture, some of which may have divided many times, some rarely.

You might think that if the Hayflick theory is correct, we'd run out of immune cells long before our allotted lifespan. Blood cells are forming and dying all the time. The average adult has billions of blood cells, including an estimated 75 billion white cells. There are 1,000 red cells for every one or two white cells in the blood. If you want your mind to be boggled, consider this: the blood cells in your body travel through more than 60,000 miles of small blood vessels, and a drop of your blood contains 5,000 to 10,000 white cells and five million red cells. One-third of white cells are lymphocytes, or T cells and B cells, which reproduce themselves whenever the body needs defending. Only a few of them live for long. But we don't run out of blood cells. The supply lasts as long as other body cells because they are derived from stem cells in the bone marrow. Whole sub-populations of blood cells come from each stem cell.

As we reach old age, the reproductive capacity of stem cells runs down. Fewer of them are still able to give rise to blood cells. Processes of aging, such as the hair going gray, are sometimes speeded up in people who have had bone marrow radiation (for example, prior to bone marrow transplant), which destroys their stem cells. But for most people in old age, enough stem cells remain to do the job. Studies indicate that the number of B cells in 80- and 90-year-olds has not decreased and that there are normal levels of antibodies circulating in their blood. However, some doctors have found that when a germ is encountered and more antibodies are called for, the old person's immune system takes longer to make the required antibodies. Doctors have found that sometimes aged patients will make no antibodies at all, if they are given an injection to immunize them against a disease.

Some studies have shown that old people have lower than average numbers of T helper cells and natural killer cells. The lower number of the latter may help explain the increased risk of cancer, since these cells go after tumor cells. Experiments in the 1970s showed that skin tests to determine the strength of a person's immune response, when given to people over the age of 80, could almost be used as a predictor of how much longer they would live. People who had no response to tests with the substances were at high risk of dying within the next two years. The death rate in that group of people was 80 per cent, compared with 35 per cent for the group who had reacted to two or more of the test substances.

The thymus gland, which is vital to the development of

T cells, peaks in size early in the teen years and from then on shrinks; by old age it is merely a remnant. In studies with mice, researchers found that if they replaced the thymus of a young animal with an old thymus, the immune system was almost as deficient as if they had left the mouse without a thymus at all. A few scientists have suggested that the thymus itself is the body's biological clock, setting the upper limit of human lifespan. As it shrinks, fewer educated T cells emerge. Helper T cells are the pivotal cells on which immune responses depend; as their numbers decline, the whole system is diminished. Furthermore, spleen and lymph nodes, other organs that make up the immune system, also become smaller. Studies have shown that old T cells multiply less rapidly and produce less interleukin-2, a growth stimulator. And cytotoxic T cells are less effective killers.

Some doctors have said that the immune system plays an important part in the aging process of the whole individual. Mankind is forever looking for the fountain of youth. We support huge industries devoted to products that are supposed to rid us of wrinkles, corset our bodies in youthful shapes, or restore our vigor. Often promoters twist or exaggerate a scientific finding known to the public to support the marvels they say their products will perform. We can expect that as scientists unravel the link between age and the immune system, we'll be offered by pseudo-scientists and companies all sorts of dubious products or treatments that are supposed to keep our immune systems young. We will need to be wary. It is easy to be taken in and at best waste our money, or at worst do ourselves harm.

For 30 years buyers have been attracted by a so-called youth restorer, devised by Rumanian doctor Ana Aslan. Dr. Aslan claimed it slows the aging process. Chemical analysis has shown it to be a mild anti-depressant. Some doctors say this may explain why some people who have taken it have claimed to feel younger and better. But if depression can, as a number of studies have shown, damp down the immune system, there might be a grain of truth in Dr. Aslan's claim, although no other studies of the product have confirmed it. In any case, elderly people are not all suffering depression.

Enough evidence to link the immune system with at least some of the aging processes has accumulated to spark tests in animals of different ways to prevent the loss of — or restore — immune responses. Immune cells from young animals have been transplanted into old ones. Scientists have also tried transplanting spleens, lymph nodes, thymus glands, and bone marrow. There have been hints of promise in a few cases. Some transplants prevented auto-immune diseases in some ancient mice. But for the most part, such experimental transplants have had no effect on the length of life of normal-aged animals.

Enzymes and hormones, such as hormones produced by the thymus gland, have also been tried as methods of rejuvenating the immune system. Most have been used only in animals. At least one researcher in the U.S. has reported interesting results in one breed of mice. There was hope among scientists initially that thymus hormones might help cancer patients fight their disease, but no thrilling results have been reported so far.

But in Japan there is interest in the effects on the immune system of a group of enzymes, known as Q because they are related to quinone, a compound found in the body in several organs. Researchers had noted that Q is lacking in the elderly. The substances have previously been used as a drug for certain heart conditions. But now, in studies with mice, researchers report indications that Q may improve the effectiveness of B cells, thus protecting the mice from viruses and possibly from tumors.

In other studies, researchers are investigating products produced by T cells during an immune response. One tantalizing product is called interleukin-2. It is a growth factor needed by T cells to make them reproduce. Researchers who tested it in aged mice found that it helps restore the immune system. Interleukin-2 is also being used as a new method of cancer treatment (see Chapter Eight) and appears able to turn certain lymphocytes into powerful killers of cancer cells.

Another intriguing substance under investigation — but a long way yet from use in people — is called DHEA, standing for the tongue-twisting name dehydroepiandrosterone. It is found in high levels in the blood of babies before birth, then drops out of sight until puberty when it rises again. It remains high in young adults, then disappears again. Scientists have puzzled over whether it has a role in the aging process. But it has proved difficult to study. It delays immune deficits in a breed of mice prone to them, but DHEA is different in mice and man: in mice, the levels don't drop with age. Too little is understood to know if it will ever be safe to give it to people, much less whether it will do them any good.

In Israel, at the Weizmann Institute, scientists have developed a substance that appears capable of improving the immune response in old mice and in immune cells obtained from elderly people and grown in the laboratory. In old age, cells and tissues lose fluid and become more rigid. The substance, given as a diet supplement, holds promise of restoring to normal the outer coverings of immune cells and also brain cells. Called AL 721, it is a mixture of lipids or fats. This is significant, for cell membranes are made largely of lipids, and scientists say that immune system malfunctions are often associated with abnormal outer membranes on immune cells. The mixture is undergoing tests in Israel and the United States.

Elderly people appear to have normal levels of B cells, yet sometimes the antibodies they produce don't seem effective — perhaps because in old age they can't reach their targets. Ordinarily, antibodies, as well as circulating in the blood and lymph, can reach tissue not in direct contact with body fluids by being passed from one cell to another. Cells use receptors, molecules on their surface, to hand over antibodies to neighbor cells. Recently, at the Veterans' Administration Medical Center in San Francisco, scientists have found that aging brings a decrease in receptors by which IgA antibodies travel in the liver. In effect, front-line defenders are cut off from reaching parts of the organ. Scientists suspect that it may happen in other regions of the body, too. It may help explain why elderly folk are more prone to intestinal diseases. The finding also helps solve a puzzle. Scientists had found that IgA antibodies did not decrease in the blood with age but that they did fall in the intestinal tract. Ordinarily, a large amount of IgA is passed through the liver into the bile, and from there is transported to the intestines. Six times less IgA passes through the liver in old rats than in young rats.

Spleen cells from old mice were 10 times less able to mount an immune attack on tumor cells than spleen cells from young mice in a University of Chicago study. Scientists measured the results when they put the different age spleen cells with tumor cells in cultures in the laboratory. But, oddly, they also found that if they crowded the old cells, tightly packing them in the cultures, they killed tumor cells almost equally as well as young cells. It has made them wonder if it may some day be possible to treat cancer in old people by packing their blood with white cells geared to attack tumor cells. So far they are only able to say that it is possible in laboratory dishes to reverse age-related loss of protection against tumors. They can't predict if it will work in the body.

On the other side of the see-saw, immune systems of old people produce more antibodies against "self" — auto-antibodies. These are found in increasing numbers as age increases. Auto-antibodies are made against regular antibodies, the two particles binding together and circulating in the blood. Some doctors say that these may pile up in the kidney or other tissues and start up a low level of chronic disease that contributes indirectly to overall aging.

In arthritis, auto-antibodies produced against a person's IgG antibodies are called rheumatoid factor. Studies have shown young, healthy people may have the factor and it increases with age. In people over the age of 70, levels of rheumatoid factor are significantly higher than in people in their 20s. At the University of New Mexico, scientists found that both T cells and B cells in old people with the factor were abnormal. Ironically, old B cells appeared less capable of producing antibodies, so the helper T cells, which tell the B cells to produce them, were overly active, working harder to drive the B cells. That may partly explain why the normal balance between T helper cells and T suppressor cells may be off kilter in people with arthritis. In addition, when the scientists grew cells from old people in the laboratory, the cells if stimulated into activity, produced a lot more rheumatoid factor than similar cells from the young. Having the factor, however, does not always mean a person has or will develop arthritis. But it is involved in inflammation in arthritic joints.

According to some scientists, it is almost inevitable that antibodies against self will crop up over the years. The immune system may be intentionally weakened in advanced years to help prevent the development of auto-immune diseases. Others suggest that the cause originates in the brain: brain cells die off and cannot be replaced with new cells. Cells of the central nervous system, during youth, lose the ability to reproduce. As understanding of the links between the brain and the immune system increases, it is becoming clear that a decrease in certain brain cells that produce chemical messages normally relayed to immune cells might affect body defenses. Studies in both people and animals have found decreased amounts of brain chemicals with age. Parkinson's disease, for example, which involves a lack of the brain chemical dopamine, is primarily a disease of older people. Parkinson's patients treated for long periods with a replacement dopamine (levodopa) have been found to live longer than untreated patients. Dopamine is known to act on the immune system.

In the elderly, one branch of the immune system — what doctors call the mucosal immune system — remains strong, according to researchers at Queen's University in Kingston, Ontario. This protective mechanism, found in the digestive tract, the respiratory system, and the genito-urinary tract, is separate from the general immune system; it might be thought of as the local police, with the general system being the national army. The discovery that the mucosal system shows no sign of weakening with age — at least in animals — has led to the suggestion that vaccinations for the elderly, such as flu shots, should be given by mouth rather than by injection. An immune response, triggered by the vaccine, would be made by white cells of the mucosal system; in particular, those old people who can make no antibodies when given conventional flu shots might benefit. The idea is being tested in a group of such people in Kingston.

There seems to be one common finding in virtually every experiment designed to discover if ways can be found to lengthen life by bolstering the immune system: if the animal loses weight, there are improvements in immune responses. From information gathered by insurance companies and in population studies, it is known that people who live the longest tend to be those who were lean in their twenties and gained only a little weight in middle age. Studies in rats and mice put on restricted diets have shown there is significant improvement in immune responses and a decrease in production of auto-antibodies. One breed of fat mouse, which normally has a very short life, outlives even normal mice if put on a diet to lose weight, even though with the weight loss they remain much fatter and heavier than ordinary mice.

So far, doctors simply don't know enough to tell people that being slim is good for their immune systems, although it may be a wise idea for many reasons related to health. They do know that malnourishment is extremely detrimental to body defenses, making people fall prey to all sorts of diseases. Until much more is learned, eating sensibly and cutting down a bit as one becomes less active with age seems the best course to take to help your immune system retain its remarkably fine balance. But it is fairly safe to predict that medical science will eventually find the way to give immune systems a drink from the fountain of youth and help people stay healthy for 100 years.

SEX DIFFERENCES

In many species, including humans, females live longer than males. In countries like Canada, the gap is widening. Fifty years or so ago, Canadian women, on average, lived only two years longer than men. The life expectancy in the 1930s was 62 years for women, 60 years for men. Today the difference is seven years, with men having a life expectancy of only 72 years to women's 79. There undoubtedly are a variety of causes for the difference, with the list encompassing employment, drinking and smoking, and heart disease. But a number of doctors are coming to believe that sex hormones and their effect on the immune system might be a bigger factor than ever before realized.

In general, females produce more antibodies than males, indicating a more effective humoral or B cell line of defense. Furthermore, women tend to reject organ transplants more readily than men, one indication of a vigorous cell-mediated or T cell line of defense.

You might think it should be the other way around. Women, after all, are designed for pregnancy, and a fetus, like a transplanted organ, is formed of cells and tissue different from the mother. Why, if a woman's immune system is so good at detecting that a transplant is foreign, does she not reject her baby? The fact that the baby is not rejected in the vast majority of cases seems to fly in the face of the most fundamental law of the immune system: get rid of whatever is not "self." Cells of the fetus carry molecules inherited from the father, which are the all-important human leukocyte antigens. They should set off in the mother a catastrophic attack on the child.

But Nature is wonderfully ingenious. A whole bag of tricks is available to protect the new life. We'll get to that in more detail a bit later. For the moment, let's consider the woman. During pregnancy, turning off her immune system entirely would be hazardous both to her and the baby. They'd have no protection against germs. Yet, for the sake of the fetus, it is essential that the mother's defenses can be readily tuned, suppressing them as well as boosting them, as required. Scientists have found a number of factors involved in this fine-tuning.

Researchers at the U.S. National Cancer Institute discovered in the urine of pregnant women a protein that is a powerful suppressor of immune responses. It is called uromodulin and acts on T cells and macrophages. It does not, however, affect B cells, the antibody producers. One kind of antibodies, IgG, can cross from the mother to the child and will provide protection against germs for the baby not only before birth, but also in the early months of life before the infant can begin producing its own antibodies. Other proteins found in pregnant women also show evidence of reducing immune responses.

On the other side of the coin, the female hormone, estrogen, can boost a certain immune responsiveness. It is possible that one job of female hormones is to counter immune suppression caused by pregnancy and restore the normal balance. Estrogen and progesterone act on macrophages and make them produce more of the proteins collectively known as interleukin-1, an essential ingredient in the process of T cell reproduction.

Boston researchers have found that interleukin-1 increases in women at the time of ovulation, when an egg is released. At that time, female sex hormones increase, accounting at least for part of the increase in interleukin-1. Incidentally, interleukin-1 raises body temperature, explaining why a woman can determine her fertile phase by taking her temperature during her monthly cycle.

Throughout pregnancy, antibodies and other immune components rise and fall dramatically at certain times, indicating that there is an incredibly complex pattern of shifts in defense mechanisms acting to protect the fetus. One Rockefeller University researcher has said: "I think that females may have developed a built-in monitoring system that both enables the fetus to survive, yet locates and destroys other foreign substances. Speaking broadly, the female immune system seems to be more finely tuned than the male." That would explain the paradox in women of heightened transplant rejection and pregnancy.

Studies have shown that male sex hormones, androgens, can suppress immune response. Injected into chick embryos, they prevented the chicks from producing antibodies. Injected into rats with skin grafts, they delayed rejection of the new foreign skin. They also reduce resistance to infections. Some scientists say male sex hormones are one reason men are more susceptible than women to infectious diseases. There is, of course, a great variation among men in their degree of susceptibility to infectious diseases. But there is also a difference from one man to another in how androgens act on the body. Some men have heavy beard growth, for example, while others do not. To add to the complexity, androgens can be converted into estrogen in the body.

In mice, according to some studies, it's not healthy to be macho. The animals that were most sensitive to androgens were the weakest immunologically. They produced lower levels of antibodies and were less able to build a defense against germs or other antigens. They were not only feebler than female mice but also than other males not as strongly affected by androgens.

But it is not always a blessing to have a potent immune system. Women are far more likely to develop certain autoimmune diseases, such as lupus. Some research suggests that estrogen slows down activity of suppressor T cells, which shut down antibody manufacture by B cells. Ordinarily, if certain B cells were producing unwanted antibodies that attack normal tissue, suppressor T cells would step in and close down production. When they don't do that, autoimmune disease can take hold. The sex hormones appear to have a profound effect on such diseases. In many cases of lupus, for example, the symptoms develop at puberty and fade away at menopause. Some women develop lupus for the first time soon after starting on the birth control pill. Estrogen in the pill may, as one doctor says, "prime the immune system like a pump"; in those women prone to lupus, an overabundance of antibodies is produced.

But it's not all that straightforward, because sometimes estrogen suppresses the immune response. Some women with arthritis find their symptoms ease when they begin taking birth control pills. In fact, estrogens and androgens have been reported both to stimulate and suppress the immune system. Both men and women normally have some of the hormones of the opposite sex. Some scientists say it depends on the ratio of estrogen to androgen whether the sex hormones pump up or deflate body defenses. Studies have shown that women with lupus have very low, or not detectable, levels of male hormones. In effect, they may have super female immune systems that tip them over into auto-immune disease. Sex hormones also affect the thymus gland, which is so crucial in making T cells into competent warriors. At puberty, when sex hormones begin to course through the body, the thymus starts to shrivel. It is known that the hormones have much to do with this decline. Researchers have shown that castration in animals will make the thymus enlarge instead of shrink. It is, needless to say, a disastrous way of improving the immune system. Conversely, if they remove the thymus of a mouse a few days after birth, reproductive organs, such as ovaries, will be attacked by lymphocytes, and levels of sex hormones will be very low.

An enormous amount is still to be learned about the interactions of body hormones, including sex hormones, and the immune system. But, considering that only a generation ago doctors did not know about any connection between reproduction and the immune system, we've come a long way.

Already scientists are devising ways to use the immune system to overcome infertility, or to produce contraceptives. A vaccine to prevent pregnancy is already being tested in Australia, as part of a multi-country program sponsored by the World Health Organization. Testing began in a small group of women in February 1986. The vaccine immunizes a woman against a hormone called human chorionic gonadotropin (HCG), which is produced soon after conception and acts on the ovaries to maintain pregnancy. The vaccine is made with a synthetic copy of part of the hormone. Other vaccines to prevent pregnancy are also being investigated. In Scotland, scientists have reported the prospect of two types of vaccines: one to produce antibodies to a covering of the egg and the other to produce antibodies to sperm.

On the egg, the antibodies would block sites where sperm attach to an egg as they try to gain entrance in order to fertilize the egg. Such antibodies are known to be produced by some women and to be a cause of some instances of involuntary infertility. They have no effect on the woman's monthly cycle or sexual behavior, and some experts consider such vaccines the most promising advances in contraception in years.

Antibodies against sperm are normally not produced. It would seem that they would be; sperm, after all, is made up of foreign cells entering the woman's body. But sperm hide under a protective coating provided in semen. If that coating is washed off and sperm is mixed with a woman's white cells, the sperm is quickly attacked; it is left alone if the coating is kept on.

But in some cases, the woman's white cells see through the sperm's disguise. At Harvard Medical School, researchers studying infertility determined that immune cells in some women attack their husbands' sperm and that this may be the reason the women are unable to get pregnant. In one study, they found that this was the case in five out of 14 women undergoing tests to determine the cause of their infertility. White cells in blood taken from the women and mixed with the sperm reacted against the sperm. About 15 per cent of the couples in North America who want families are infertile, and in some cases no physical reason can be found. The immune system could be the cause in at least a portion of these cases. Doctors have discovered that sperm antibodies produced by a woman will sometimes fade away if her immune system is not repeatedly exposed to sperm. The doctors may advise a couple to use condoms for a while to allow time for the antibodies to vanish; then conception may be possible.

It is also possible, although rare, for a man to make antibodies against his own sperm. Some unknown factor leads the immune system to make a mistake and the auto-immune condition occurs. From studies of sperm antibodies, doctors may be able both to prevent and cause infertility. When birth control is the goal, a vaccine to create antibodies against sperm might be used, just as a measles vaccine creates antibodies against a measles virus. Antibodies against the sperm antibodies may rescue the sperm and thus help overcome infertility caused by unwanted antibodies against sperm.

In some instances, miscarriages also may be the fault of the immune system. In certain women, the measures the body takes to prevent the fetus from being rejected may fail. Strange as it seems, doctors can use white cells from the father to increase protection of the fetus. In England, among 400 women who had repeatedly miscarried, one in three was able to give birth successfully after injections of the father's white cells. This treatment to preserve pregnancy is being tested in 26 medical centers in Europe and the United States and is expected to be tried in Canada soon. One would think that white cells from the father would make the mother's immune system more aware of the foreign character of the fetus. Paradoxically, that is not what happens.

The miracle of pregnancy is that a fetus is usually safe from the mother's immune cells. The mother's defense cells are quite able to identify her baby as foreign to herself. If, for instance, a bit of skin from the baby was grafted onto the mother immediately after birth, the skin would be rapidly and viciously attacked.

Yet, incredibly, the greater the difference between the self antigens of mother and baby before birth, the better the chance the child will be healthy. When mother and father have human leukocyte antigen molecules that are too much alike (as might be the case in close relatives or in a couple that would be a good match for a transplant), the baby suffers. The size of the placenta, the organ that nourishes the fetus in the womb, is affected by the difference between mother and child. The greater the difference, the larger the placenta. The T cells in the mother that recognize the fetus as foreign produce a growth factor hormone that helps both the placenta and the fetus to grow. The father's cells also stimulate the mother's antibody production, including antibodies that "hide" the fetus.

The placenta is the organ through which oxygen and nutrients pass from the mother to the fetus. Here an immune battle takes place: A layer of tissue that is formed of fetal cells, called the trophoblast, is under relentless attack. But it is far from defenseless against the mother's warriors. It deliberately provokes production of antibodies by the mother — but not antibodies that will harm the fetus. Quite the opposite. They cuddle up to fetal cells and make them invisible to maternal immune cells that could destroy them. Doctors call these protective antibodies enhancing antibodies because they increase fetal safety.

Antibodies from the mother that will act against germs are let through the barrier between the mother's blood and the baby's, but most of the destructive maternal antibodies against fetal antigens are effectively kept out. Should some get through, the trophoblast uses other strategy. It sheds, into the womb, decoy antigens or cells for the antibodies to latch onto, diverting them from the baby. The trophoblast can also produce molecules that will attract those cells in the mother that suppress the immune attack, drawing them to the site to halt any damage. At McMaster University in Hamilton, Ontario, doctors are testing this substance in women who have had miscarriages, in an attempt to bring about a successful pregnancy.

Meantime, the fetus is also taking part in its own defense. As soon as the fertilized egg is implanted in the womb, it sends out signals telling the mother's immune system not to attack. Cells that suppress the mother's immune system are found in the lining of the uterus; these are the cells that are boosted by immunization with the father's white cells. Scientists have found these suppressor cells, in animals, are so powerful that they can maintain pregnancies that nature would never otherwise allow to continue; for example, a zebra or a donkey born to horse mares.

The fetus also produces substances, such as alphafeto-protein, that suppress the T cells in the mother that would recognize and attack fetal cells. The baby's own T cells also seem able to suppress the mother's T cells. Researchers have found that if T cells from a mother and her newborn are mixed together in a culture dish, the T cells that become active and reproduce are 95 per cent baby cells. Ordinarily, if two people's T cells are mixed, those that are stimulated into action are half from one person, half from the other.

Many of the remarkable measures that have developed to ensure the survival of a fetus starting existence in what is potentially an awesomely hostile environment are teaching researchers lessons that may in future help fight cancer. Perhaps tumors use the same tricks as a fetus to hide from attacks. Doctors are discovering how to improve protection for an unborn baby by preventing a possible attack on it by immune cells. They may be able to flip the coin and remove protection from tumor cells so that they cannot elude an immune attack.

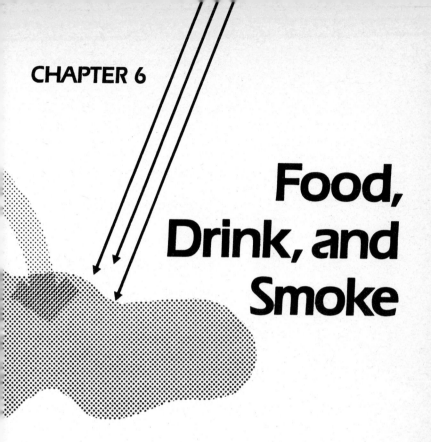

CHAPTER 6

Food, Drink, and Smoke

Among a tribe of Indian people on Vancouver Island in British Columbia, almost half have arthritis. In what has been termed an arthritis epidemic, one in six of them becomes severely crippled. This phenomenon has attracted the attention of an international team of researchers from Canada, Britain, Belgium, and the United States. The reason for the wide interest? Not simply to find ways to help the 200 members of the tribe, but also to take advantage of a rare opportunity to discover much more about the link between diet and body defenses.

For 20,000 years, salmon was the staple of the Nuu-Chaa Nulth tribe's diet. Then they switched to white man's foods. The researchers hope to find out if this change caused serious consequences to the Indians' health. If so, they will try to determine by what mechanisms particular foods have an impact on cells of the immune system. The study holds promise; within the past few months, scientists have found that fish oils, or more specifically an essential fatty acid contained in fish oils, may offer a new way to prevent damage to tissue done by misdirected immune cells in auto-immune diseases such as arthritis. Some propose that cyclosporine A, a drug being used to treat a number of other auto-immune diseases, be put in fish oil because the oil might help prevent toxic effects of the drug on kidneys on top of reducing damage done by the disease.

Only a few years ago, scientists might not have recognized the opportunity being provided by the Indians in this real-life laboratory situation. Doctors had no idea how much the efficiency of immune cells depends on fatty acids, obtained from plants, meat, and fish, and on vitamins and trace minerals. Nutrition, until recent years, was not a high priority in the world of medicine. It was generally believed that as long as people had *enough* food, their ability to combat infectious diseases was not affected. It was known that severe malnutrition, such as seen among children in poverty-stricken Third World countries, made many children helpless victims of childhood diseases. The death toll among those who caught measles, for example, was appallingly high. But that extreme degree of malnourishment was not often seen in North America or in other industrialized nations. In the western world, discoveries of nutrition's impact on health first came from research into heart disease and cancer. But immunologists deemed this outside their domain.

Today, however, new information shows that your immune system relies to a large extent for its health on what you eat.

Among the nutrients it needs are vitamins. The World Health Organization (WHO) has reported that vitamin A is vital to the immune response. Even moderate vitamin A deficiencies increase sickness due to respiratory and gastrointestinal infections. WHO studies have been conducted in children, six months to six years of age, in underdeveloped countries. Among these children, vitamin A deficiency is obvious because it causes serious eye diseases and blindness.

In one study of 27,000 of these children over two years, researchers found they were three times more likely to get infectious diseases than children getting an adequate amount of vitamin A. Tragically, the death rate among under-nourished children was four to twelve times as high as would be expected in properly fed youngsters.

The family of B vitamins are known to have a powerful effect on immune cells in several different ways, especially on the production of antibodies. One study has shown that without one kind of vitamin B, the B cells of the immune system are unable to mature to the stage at which they can produce antibodies.

Many claims for vitamin C's ability to fight off the common cold have been made, including those by Nobel prize-winner Linus Pauling, who wrote a widely publicized book about it. However, a large study at the University of Toronto, and studies elsewhere involving thousands of people, did not confirm the claim that large doses of vitamin C prevent the pesky infections. They did find, however, that people taking the vitamin suffered somewhat milder symptoms when they got colds. One study at the University of Oregon discovered that vitamin C can increase production of interferon, one of the substances cells make when they are infected with viruses.

Some practitioners recommend that AIDS patients take vitamin C supplements. It may make sense. Studies of these patients have shown they produce abnormally low amounts of interferon. Vitamin C has also been found to help prevent damage within cells caused by so-called free radicals, which are produced as cells use oxygen. Radicals can bash around inside the cells; vitamin C, along with vitamins A and E, sponge them up. Vitamin C also helps preserve the thymus and other lymph organs and increases the power of macrophages to engulf and chew up bacteria, according to other studies.

Vitamin E, as well as protecting against damage from free radicals, also plays a role in wound healing, a process that involves immune cells. The vitamin helps reduce inflammation. In 1955, the first studies of vitamin E's effects on the immune system were observed in rabbits. Given supplements of the vitamin, the rabbits more quickly produced antibodies to typhoid vaccine and other toxins.

University of Colorado studies in the 1970s found that in mice, the vitamin increased the proliferation of antibody-producing B cells. It also was established that B cells shifted production of antibodies from IgM to IgG, a more effective type of antibody. The vitamin, according to other studies, seems to enhance cooperation between T helper cells and B cells. Colorado researchers have also discovered some indications that the oily Vitamin E, incorporated into vaccines, may help prevent reactions in people hypersensitive to components of the vaccines. Several studies in poultry and mice infected with bacteria have shown that vitamin E supplements increased the effectiveness of macrophages in chewing up bacteria. It has not been found to have a booster effect on T cells, or on increasing protection against viral infections.

Trace minerals also play a part. For example, a deficiency of zinc can bring on a total immune deficiency disease. Before doctors knew the cause, the disease was usually fatal. Now it can be cured by giving patients zinc tablets. Too little zinc can cause a loss of T cells of all kinds and a shrinkage of the thymus gland. Some nutritionists have said that zinc deficiency can occur even in reasonably well-fed people because the mineral is lost from processed foods. Foods rich in zinc include meat, eggs, milk, poultry and whole grains.

Magnesium is another mineral the immune system requires to stay healthy. It is found in nuts, soybeans, whole grains, and raw leafy green vegetables. Copper is needed by the thymus gland to produce its hormones. Some studies in both people and mice have shown that a lack of copper makes infections far more severe. Still another mineral, selenium, working in concert with vitamin E, has been found to improve production of antibodies. It is obtained from seafood, chicken, garlic, whole grains, and milk. Iron is an ingredient of chemicals made by T cells. The body can absorb only a fraction of the iron you eat, but that amount can be increased if iron-rich foods, primarily meats, are eaten at the same time as foods containing vitamin C. Beef and tomatoes, for example, are a good combination.

But while your immune system can't do without vitamins and minerals, too much of any good thing can sap its vigor as well. The last thing you should do is rush out to buy stacks of food supplements to improve body defenses. Overdoses of some vitamins, such as vitamin A, can do you grievous harm, in effect poisoning you. Many people think they need extra iron. But the body stores iron and too much of it can increase the risk of bacterial and fungal infections. Some wretched bacteria need lots of iron to thrive.

The care and feeding of your immune system calls for common sense about diet. You need to eat a wide variety of foods to supply the different substances. If you fear your eating habits may be the reason you catch frequent colds or other germs, discuss your diet with your doctor or a qualified nutritionist. There is little doubt that a poor diet weakens immune responses. But self-doctoring by indiscriminately gobbling down supplements can make your immune cells throw up their hands in dismay.

In Newfoundland, a quarter of the children examined in one large study were found to have deficient immune systems. Specialists there say it is the direct result of faulty nutrition. The children, typically, drink only a quarter of the milk drunk by children in other parts of Canada; fresh vegetables are expensive and scarce and not even very fresh when they arrive at outpost villages; and, surprisingly, families there eat little fish. A study at Memorial University established that undernourished children in St. John's have more infectious diseases and are sick longer with them. Those sick enough to go to hospital spend 30 per cent longer in hospital than other, well-nourished children before they recover. Studies in Texas have shown that people eating diets too low in protein do not react normally to skin tests when being checked for tuberculosis. But put them on good diets and their immune responses are restored. Moderate to severe malnutrition typically results in reduced levels of T cells. Although B cells may be normal in numbers, without enough helper T cells they are unable to produce a good supply of antibodies. Adequate protein in the diet is essential to the production of antibodies. If you don't give your body defenses the nutrients they need to do their jobs, germs that gain entry to the body might meet with little resistance.

Much controversy rages around the connection between auto-immune diseases and diet. At some centers, it is claimed that certain foods make symptoms of arthritis worse and that by having patients fast and follow special diets, their immune systems become more balanced and their disease abates. Other doctors dismiss the claims as hogwash. As scientists steadily winkle out facts, they find changed food patterns a possible explanation for the improvement in some select patients with an auto-immune disease such as arthritis. It may have to do with the kind of essential fatty acids in diet. And some of these provocative findings suggest there there is a direct connection between diet and heart disease, too.

The story is complex and will eventually take us back to the British Columbia Indians. It begins with research into substances in the body that regulate many body functions. Among them are prostaglandins, an amazingly versatile family of hormone-like substances found in small quantities in virtually all body organs, especially the pancreas, lungs, and liver. Discovered in the 1930s, the substances were given their name — an inappropriate one as it turned out — because they were thought to come only from the prostate gland, a part of the male reproductive system. Investigation into prostaglandins revealed that they were made from certain fatty acids. Clearly, here was a link to diet, because the human body cannot make all fatty acids and must get some of them from food. They are called "essential fatty acids." The most important essential fatty acid, which is the kind required by the body to make prostaglandins, is linoleic acid, which primarily comes from plants. It is in polyunsaturated fats found in vegetable oils.

Studies of prostaglandins began to lead researchers to the immune system. They focused on one species of mice that spontaneously develops a condition similar to severe lupus and affecting the whole T cell network, making the animals unable to reject transplants of any kind of tissue. Giving these mice one kind of prostaglandin returned the whole immune system to normal. Giving them linoleic acid, which their bodies could turn into prostaglandin, prevented the condition from developing. Prostaglandin could also clear up an arthritis-like condition in rats.

When rats, from the day they were weaned, were fed a diet free of all fats, they were observed to grow poorly, lose their hair and weight, have enlarged lymph nodes and spleens, develop eczema on their skins, and have low levels of T cells. The whole syndrome could be turned around by feeding them essential fatty acids. On the other hand, different studies found that diets very high in fats brought about a speedy shrinking of the thymus, the gland that is vital to T cell development.

From patients who spent long periods in hospital, unable to eat and fed by means of intravenous fluids, doctors learned that any number of conditions that could be traced back to diminished immune cells could arise as a result of malnutrition, in particular a shortage of essential fatty acids. (Today, patients who can't eat for long periods are given vastly more nutritious fluids.) Patients deprived of essential fatty acids produced an abnormal number of antibodies. Such patients also had an imbalance of T cells, with a significant loss of suppressor cells. A similar imbalance is frequently seen in auto-immune diseases.

Another essential fatty acid, primarily obtained from meat, although the body can make it from linoleic acid, is required to allow the body to produce another family of substances called leukotrienes, made by white blood cells. Both prostaglandins and leukotrienes are produced at the site of injuries. They also play a part in inflammation in arthritic joints. Some prostaglandins increase inflammation and others, which act like anti-inflammatory drugs, such as Aspirin, cool it down. Immune cells swarm to the site of infection, called in by signals from leukotrienes. The latter also act on immune cells in a number of different ways, and there is much to learn about them yet. One kind of leukotriene can bring on symptoms of asthma and arthritis.

Fish oils contain a different kind of essential fatty acid, called eicosapentaenoic acid. Studies are showing that it reduces the inflammatory process. Harvard Medical School researchers found that the acid decreased the release of leukotrienes. They studied the process in healthy young men who took fish oil supplements for six weeks. In other studies, in California, people with arthritis who ate a high fish diet, thus reducing the quantity of leukotrienes, suffered fewer inflammatory symptoms in their joints.

The team studying the British Columbia Indians are focusing sharply on leukotrienes and prostaglandins. "If those substances get out of balance, there's hell to pay," says one Canadian team member. "If there is too much or too little, the consequences for health are profound." It may be that by giving up the traditional diet, high in fish fatty acid, the tribe members have suffered an imbalance causing the epidemic of arthritis. It may be that the Indians, and possibly other people with arthritis, cannot make a substance to curb production of leukotrienes themselves and must get it from fish.

Heart disease may involve a similar mechanism. High cholesterol levels in the blood have long been linked to an increased risk of heart disease. Now researchers have found that when cholesterol is in the early stages of causing hardening of the arteries, macrophages stick to the walls of the blood vessels, adding to the blockage. What makes them stick there? Leukotrienes. And fish oil fatty acids prevent the macrophages from adhering. The findings suggest then, that by a change of diet, immune cells can be changed; this in turn may help prevent heart disease as well as auto-immune disease.

Heart disease may involved a similar mechanism. High cholesterol levels in the blood have long been linked to an increased risk of heart disease. Now researchers have found that when cholesterol is in the early stages of causing hardening of the arteries, macrophages stick to the walls of the blood vessels, adding to the blockage. What makes them stick there? Leukotrinnes. And fish oil fatty acids prevent the macrophages from adhering. The findings suggest then, that by a change of diet, immune cells can be changed; this in turn may prevent heart disease as well as auto-immune disease.

There is much more to be learned, however, before doctors will know which patients should be advised to alter their diets to any great extent. Macrophage activity in blood vessels is not all bad. Macrophages may play a part in preventing blood clots, which can also be a cause of blockage in heart arteries.

Other clues about the link between essential fatty acids and auto-immune disease have been uncovered by the study of diabetes. People with diabetes are often more susceptible to infectious diseases. Evidence is accumulating that a deficiency in essential fatty acids, or in the way they are turned into prostaglandins and leukotrienes, may be the cause. A study at the University of Minnesota has found that vegetarians may be at less risk of developing diabetes. Looking at more than 25,000 Seventh Day Adventists who are vegetarians, the researchers found they had less than half the general population's risk of diabetes.

In general, diet in North America is too heavy in fats. Such a diet, by its effects on the thymus gland, leads to a shortage of effective T cells. Doctors advise cutting back a bit so that fats make up less than a third of calories consumed. But they also suggest that people eat different kinds of fats: polyunsaturated fats such as fish and corn oil, mono-unsaturated fats like olive oil, and saturated fats found in meat and dairy products.

Researchers have learned that people who find certain foods bring about mood changes, making them irritable, anxious, or depressed, sometimes experience marked changes in the immune system when they eat those foods. In a University of Chicago study, 16 of 23 subjects with mea-surable mood changes resulting from foods had significantly lower levels of complement in their blood (the family of chemicals that act with antibodies to kill invaders). The unpleasant emotions such people feel may be a message from their immune cells trying to tell them a particular food isn't doing the cells any good. Brain chemicals that modify moods can affect immune cells (see Chapter Four, on stress). Sugar, milk, wheat, corn, and chocolate are commonly among the foods people say change their moods, even though they do not have allergic reactions to them.

Some doctors say that food allergies are actually quite rare. They limit the meaning of allergy to conditions brought about by IgE antibodies. But others say food sensitivities can cause symptoms by affecting T cells, the chemicals they make (lymphokines), antibodies, complement, and prostaglandins. The result may be migraine headaches, plugged ears or a ringing in the ears, irritable bowel syndrome, or an array of other symptoms for which no cause can be found. Elim-inating suspect foods from the diet to see if the symptoms go away is the usual way of making the diagnosis.

As you can see, your mouth is a doorway to your immune system. Through it you may be able to help keep your white cells on their toes or deal them a staggering blow. Food isn't the only thing that creates problems, however. Alcohol and smoking may give body defenses a double whammy.

It is possible that alcohol sets off a kind of auto-immune disease in the liver. Heavy alcohol consumption has long been known to lead to inflammation and cirrhosis of the liver. Scientists at the University of California in San Francisco have found that alcohol causes liver cells to attract white blood cells. The liver is your body's detoxification center. Doctors already knew that large numbers of immune cells could be found in damaged and inflamed livers of people who drank heavily. Immune cells are called in to any site of tissue injury or damage. But now they see something new. The evidence indicates that liver cells, as soon as they have absorbed alcohol, send out a message that calls in the defense troops; these defending white cells actually do the damage, attacking the liver.

Cigarette smoking has many impacts on immune cells. A U.S. Surgeon General's report on smoking summed up a number of studies indicating an impairment in immune responses in smokers. Macrophages in these people were less able to show foreign material to T cells and to produce chemicals that are crucial both in destruction of bacteria and in communicating with other immune cells. A component of smoke, nitrogen oxide, reduces resistance to viral infections, possibly by lessening production of interferon, the report said. Other studies indicated that smoking lessens production of antibodies and that smokers are more susceptible during outbreaks of influenza. Researchers found that components of cigarette smoke reduced the number of B cells in the spleen.

Scientists have discovered that babies born to women who smoke during pregnancy tend to weigh less; the reason may be that the fetus is less able to protect itself against attacks from the mother's immune cells. One way it does this is to stimulate the mother's body to produce protective antibodies. But smoking mothers are less able to produce antibodies.

In Chicago, scientists have found indications that use of marijuana can disrupt the immune system and leave users more vulnerable to colds and other infections. They found the drug changes the outer covering of T cells and also affects production of prostaglandins. Studies in guinea pigs showed that marijuana made the animals more susceptible to herpes, and American investigators have also suggested the drug may make matters worse for people with other viral infections, including AIDS.

Searching for ways to help strengthen the immune system, doctors have found one of the easiest methods may be exercise. It sounds as if they're suggesting we coax our immune cells into doing sit-ups and push-ups, doesn't it? How on earth could we do that? It turns out that when people run or exercise vigorously, the levels of T cells in their bloodstreams rise. At the University of Michigan, scientists noted that people who exercise for an hour produce a chemical in their blood similar to substances produced when one has an infection and fever. Interleukin-1 is responsible for fever; apparently exercise stimulated the production of this immune system product. Blood taken from the exercisers and injected into rats caused the same fever and blood changes, including a decrease in iron that would be seen in an infection in the animals. Higher temperatures and a drop in iron in the blood are hostile conditions for bacteria. Any of those trouble-makers hanging around at that moment might suddenly find the cards stacked against them.

But beware of exercising your immune system into exhaustion. Researchers at the University of New Mexico have reported that excessive exercise — such as a two-hour bicycle road race — results in lowered levels of antibodies, possibly leaving you vulnerable to infections. It only lasts a short while, however; antibody levels return to normal within a day. Researchers admit that the effects on the immune system could be caused by stress, not pedaling.

Overfeeding the body — in man or mouse — reduces its ability to fight off infections, according to the University of Toronto's Dr. Bernhard Cinader. He says that restricting calories fed to mice makes their immune systems more effective. But, he adds, genetic differences between strains of mice or between individuals, play a key part in the way diet affects the immune system; not enough is known yet to make general recommendations concerning the best nutrition for body defense.

All in all, it appears that keeping yourself fit and eating a nutritious, but not fattening, diet make sense for more reasons than you might have thought. In effect, they keep your immune system troops in top fighting form.

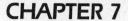

CHAPTER 7

Transplants and Transfusions

Frankenstein, the fictional medical student dreamed up in 1818 by novelist Mary Shelley, created a monster by putting together human parts obtained from cemeteries. At the time, no doubt, the idea of using parts from the dead to give new life was utterly shocking. Yet 149 years later, a South African dentist was to refer to himself jokingly as the "new Frankenstein" creation. In December 1967, Louis Washkansky was the first person to be given a heart transplant, when his own failing one was replaced with the heart of a 24-year-old killed in a traffic accident.

At that time, though the idea of replacing a person's heart — the organ long associated with love and emotions —

was startling, transplants of other kinds had become relatively common in many medical centers.

Kidneys were being transplanted with regularity. The first kidney transplant had been performed in 1955 in Boston, where Richard Harrick was successfully given a kidney from his twin brother. Early in the century, an Austrian eye specialist, Eduard Zirm, had transplanted corneas — the transparent covering of the pupil in the front of the eye — into the eyes of patients. The first such transplant was performed in 1902 by Dr. Zirm on a workman whose own eyes had been burned with lye; his sight was restored when he received the corneas of a dead 11-year-old boy.

Bone marrow transplants were also sometimes success-ful. The first one was done in Paris by Dr. Georges Mathe, in 1963, to treat a 26-year-old patient with leukemia, cancer of blood cells. In that same year, the first lung transplant was attempted and failed. The patient, an American, was a convicted murderer. And in Colorado, Dr. Thomas Starzl was pioneering in liver transplants.

From the beginning, kidney transplants were the most successful. In about half the cases, the new kidney began working as if it had always been there, enabling the patient to live a quite normal life. But sometimes the patient's body simply would not accept the new organ. Doctors called it "rejection." The tissue of the transplant became so damaged that the kidney had to be removed and the patient put back on treatment with an artificial kidney in a process called dialysis. In the 1950s, little was known about the immune system's T cell (cell-mediated) line of defense. Indeed, interest in research into the immune system had waned greatly with the advent of antibiotic drugs effective in treating many infectious diseases. It was believed that the prime job of the immune system was to combat infections, and once there were drugs to solve the problem, science more or less neglected the immune system itself.

But transplants sparked a new era of research into immune responses. Doctors saw that the chances of a suc-cessful kidney transplant were greater when the donor was a relative of the patient whose tissues were similar. Tests called tissue typing were developed to determine how well the tissues of two people matched. Steroid drugs and drugs used to treat cancer were found to help prevent rejection. The cancer drugs acted against immune cells because they are designed to target cells that are dividing into two, and one of the first steps in a cell-mediated immune response is for T cells to divide. But all the anti-rejection drugs knocked patients' whole immune systems out of commission, leaving them vulnerable to infections. Physicians had to learn to walk a tightrope, balancing the patient's treatment to avoid rejection, on the one hand, and infection, on the other.

Dealing with the problem became even more critical in heart transplants. Rejection of a kidney didn't mean the inevitable death of the patient. But in a heart transplant patient whose body objected strenuously to the foreign tissue, rejection meant game over. The South African dentist, whose new heart was transplanted in Capetown by Dr. Christiaan Barnard, lived only 18 days before rejection and pneumonia killed him.

While much of the world acclaimed Dr. Barnard's daring in attempting the surgical rescue of a doomed heart patient, most of the medical profession was not similarly enthralled with Dr. Barnard. In their view, he had jumped the gun. Worse, he had stolen the glory from a California medical scientist, Dr. Norman Shumway, who had done many years of research and was the true father of heart transplantation. Dr. Barnard had, for a time, studied with Dr. Shumway.

But once the floodgates were opened, medical centers everywhere, including Montreal and Toronto, hustled to join the heart transplant rush. Within the next year, 50 centers performed 100 transplants. Prematurely. With only a few exceptions, the patients didn't live long. By 1970, most of the centers had abandoned the procedure. But Dr. Shumway at Stanford University did not give up. Between 1970 and 1980, his team performed more than half of the heart transplants done in the world. From 1968 to 1984, more than 300 heart transplants were performed at his university's medical center. The surgery — itself relatively simple for a good surgeon — had never been the problem. The problem was to find ways to get around the immune response and to discover how to diagnose rejection early.

Slow, steady progress was being made. But it is unlikely the resurgence of heart transplants in the 1980s would have occurred had it not been for one odd event.

Employees of a drug company had brought back to Basel, Switzerland soil that they had dug up in Norway. They were searching for anti-microbe agents that might make new antibiotics. The soil contained a strange kind of fungus that produced a substance that didn't dissolve in water. Testing showed it wasn't particularly good as an antibiotic, but it was handed over to a researcher, Dr. Jean Borel, to find out if it had any other use. Dr. Borel, investigating its effect on the immune response and cancer, was astonished to discover that the new substance seemed to reduce cell-mediated immunity involving T cells. But it didn't kill T cells like other immune-suppressant drugs. Nor did it kill other bone marrow cells, the source of all blood cells. Other immune-suppressant drugs did, which was the reason patients given them were susceptible to infections.

The drug company had been on the verge of dropping its immunology research. Dr. Borel persuaded them otherwise; Sandoz, the drug company, named the substance cyclosporine A, and by 1979 it was available for testing. Cyclosporine A revolutionized the transplant field. Success rates for transplants of all kinds jumped. In 1983, Dr. Shumway reported that since his group had begun using it, in 1980, instances of rejection of transplanted hearts had dropped dramatically. Dr. Starzl said that before cyclosporine, liver transplants were risky at best. Afterwards, at the one-year mark, 70 per cent of such transplants were successful.

Cyclosporine was tried first in kidney transplants in 10 carefully selected centers where transplants were already showing above average success rates. The drug company reasoned that cyclosporine would have to be something special if it showed itself better than the anti-rejection drugs already being used at these top centers. The first doctor to try it anywhere was Dr. Roy Calne of Cambridge, England, in 1978. At first he judged it a poor product. His patients seemed to show more signs of kidney rejection than expected. Dr. Calne had accidentally discovered a major side-effect of the drug: given in too high doses it can cause kidney damage. It wasn't rejection of the transplants he was seeing, but drug damage that mimicked rejection. At the time, doctors didn't know that much lower doses could be used successfully. In Canada only 17 of the first 103 patients given the drug rejected their transplants, compared with 35 of a similar group of patients given the then standard therapy. In 12 Canadian centers, the success rate rose from an average of 55 per cent to 77 per cent.

The impact of the exciting reports was enormous. In Canada, heart transplant programs started up again, beginning in London, Ontario, where the University of Western Ontario's University Hospital was a key North American cyclosporine test center. Combined heart and lung transplants now could also be performed successfully, an important advance for patients whose heart disease had badly damaged their lungs or for those whose lung disease had disabled their hearts.

For the first time, the transplant of a lung alone (without the heart) had a happy outcome. In November 1983, at Toronto General Hospital, a team led by Dr. Joel Cooper performed the first lung transplant to prove a long-lasting success. Until then, no lung transplant patient had lived for a year. But Thomas Hall, 58 at the time of the operation, and at first considered too old to be a recipient, came through with flying colors. As these words are being written, more than three years later, he remains well and is able to work normally.

There are now people alive who have had more than one kind of transplant. One man, who received a heart transplant at Stanford University in 1974, was given a kidney transplant in 1985. A Texas child, Stormie Jones, six, born with a rare genetic disease that caused her to have two heart attacks, underwent heart transplant and liver transplant surgery in 1984. Her own liver was abnormal, lacking the ability to clear her body of cholesterol, the high amount of which had led to the heart attacks.

Although a major discovery, cyclosporine A is not perfect. It does not completely eliminate the risk of rejection. In particular, it does not prevent all attacks by antibodies on the blood vessels of the transplanted heart. And it causes adverse side-effects, including kidney damage in some cases, and high blood pressure, although doctors have now learned how to prevent most problems by using lower doses. As Dr. Borel and his colleagues investigated the amazing product in detail, they discovered how to modify it. Now a newer, possibly less toxic, version of the drug, called cyclosporine G, is being tested. In mid-1986, researchers in Japan announced that they had devised a new anti-rejection drug, also derived from a fungus; early testing has indicated that it may be relatively harmless to kidneys.

For scientists, the thrilling discovery of cyclosporine provided proof that it is possible to control parts of the immune system without shutting down the whole defense mechanism. That opens the door to enormous possibilities and to the promise of many new kinds of treatments. Already there is tantalizing evidence that cyclosporine can prevent development of diabetes in some people and might work against multiple sclerosis. It is dramatically effective against myasthenia gravis, the disease that killed Aristotle Onassis; doctors have found that it halts progression of the muscle-weakening disease. (See Chapter Three on auto-immune diseases.)

Cyclosporine acts on T helper cells. It is believed that it interferes with the chemical messages (possibly including interleukin-2) that cause them to multiply. As we learned in an earlier chapter, interleukin-2 is a growth factor produced by T helper cells when they encounter an antigen. Cyclosporine also halts damage by macrophages; when chemical messages are sent from T helper cells to macrophages, the drug may intercept these signals, too. Not all the complexities of exactly how the drug works are understood.

Nevertheless, it has brought about a great increase in the number and kinds of transplants. Research is under way into a wide array of transplants, from bowel to limb to Fallopian tubes. Some bowel transplants have been attempted in patients; it will take time to know how successful they will be ultimately. In California, hind legs have been transplanted from black rats to white rats and vice versa, as researchers seek to find how to transplant "packages" of tissue composed of bone, skin, muscle, blood vessels, and nerves. In Montreal, scientists brought limb transplants one step closer to humans by transplanting paws of baboons. They found the animals could use their new paws with agility in three or four weeks. In British Columbia, scientists are conducting research in sheep into the transplantation of Fallopian tubes to lead them to a possible remedy for infertility in women who cannot become pregnant because their own tubes are blocked.

While transplants of the whole pancreas or segments of

the organ have proven difficult — some 900 have been performed but less than half lasted a year — transplantation of islet cells, the cells that produce insulin in the pancreas, looks promising. Inserting them does not require major surgery and, at several centers where they are being implanted in patients, there are glimmers of success. In Toronto, at the Connaught Laboratories, Dr. Anthony Sun and a team of researchers are getting close to perfecting a way of putting islet cells inside tiny protective bubbles where immune cells can't reach them. It is even possible, that the encapsulated islet cells could be animal cells. Ordinarily the human body would reject any part of an animal far more rapidly and aggressively than a transplant from another human. But inside the tiny capsules, the islet cells would not be spotted as cells from a different species. Animal insulin works perfectly well in people. With some exceptions, most diabetics can be given insulin obtained from animals, and for many years, before genetic engineering made it possible to produce insulin in the laboratory, animals were the only source of insulin used in treatment of diabetics.

So far, transplantation of organs from animals to humans has not been possible. In the United States, in 1985, an attempt was made to transplant a baboon heart into a baby girl in the hope the new anti-rejection drug could even make transplants from animals possible. A patient's immune system recognizes foreign human tissue and puts up an objection to it, but the reaction to tissue from another species is much more violent. The baby did not survive. But immunologists say it is possible to cross, temporarily, species barriers between related animal families: fox to wolf, for example, or sheep to goat. The transplant will survive for about 60 days. Thus a baboon heart implanted in a dying patient could last long enough to keep the patient alive until a human heart was available for transplant. At present, artificial hearts have been used in some cases as the bridge, tiding the patient over. But scientists predict that some day enough will be known about the immune system that it will be possible to cross the species barrier safely and permanently.

Today, however, human donors are still needed. Paradoxically, the rising transplant success rate has created a different problem: a shortage of organs to be used for transplants. It's a world-wide problem. Donors, with the exception of those who are living relatives of a kidney patient and offer to give the patient one of their kidneys, are usually accident victims with fatal head injuries.

It's heartbreaking for a family to watch a patient in urgent need of a new heart or liver go downhill, while awaiting a donor who may not be found in time. Families know there is a proven treatment that could give the patient a strong chance for recovery and find it unbearable that accident victims who could be donors are dying virtually every day, but without doing their beloved any good, because the connection that might have linked donor and recipient is not being made. Sadly, the family of the accident victim loses out, too, say a number of people who have experienced the situation first hand. One young Ontario couple, whose small daughter was tragically struck down by ice falling from a roof as the three strolled along a street in their home town, chose to donate the child's organs for transplants; three other tots were given new chances for healthy lives. "Making the decision somehow lifted a great burden of grief from us," the child's mother said later.

The difficulty in obtaining donors does not stem from the fact that too few of the people who die have suitable organs or from public opposition to transplants. In Ontario alone, of 70,000 people who die each year, 2,000 could be donors, but only 12 per cent, 240 of them on average, become donors. In the U.S. in 1982, among 20,000 young or middle-aged persons declared brain dead, only 2,500 had their organs used in transplants. Polls have shown that 88 per cent of people approve of transplants and say they would donate. Yet too often families of a dying patient are not asked their wishes. And many people have not signed organ donor cards, pledging organs at death.

Most of us don't relish the thought of sudden death and would rather not consider the idea. But it is really no different from making out your will. If you haven't yet made your wishes known and want to do so, there are a number of mechanisms available. In most provinces, a consent form is attached to drivers' licenses. The Canadian government sends out the forms with family allowance cheques. Or, if you prefer, you can carry in your wallet a plain piece of paper stating your wishes and signed by you and your next of kin. Make sure your family or those closest to you know how you feel. Your license or the piece of paper could be overlooked or have been misplaced. Each person has the right to say what will happen to his or her body after death, but even if you have signed a card, doctors will not go against the family's wishes if they refuse to let your organs be transplanted. Not many do, but it could happen if your desire has not been discussed. Some religions, such as the Muslim faith, oppose the taking of parts, which transplant doctors say creates a global dilemma because patients in Muslim areas needing transplants require donors from the western world, while most people prefer their donation be used to help others in their own land.

In Canada and other like-minded countries, it is illegal to buy or sell human tissue for transplants. The idea of poor people selling their kidneys to the rich is abhorrent. In 1983, in Alberta, a 41-year-old man created an uproar when he advertised that he would pay $5,000 for a healthy person's kidney. The man had been on a waiting list for a long time and his frustration was understandable. Under the same circumstances, any one of us might be willing to pay. Yet the human body is too precious to barter. A donated organ is a gift beyond price, and many who have received such a gift treasure it with deep gratitude. As the wife of a Canadian artist who was given the heart of a young woman explained, "It's as if this girl's heart were kissing his soul."

But when no lifesaving donation is forthcoming, relatives become desperate. Some families have enlisted the aid of famous personalities to make the public aware of children urgently needing liver transplants. One Canadian couple, who took what a doctor calls "the celebrity route," persuaded a federal cabinet minister, the American ambassador to Canada, and hockey superstar Wayne Gretzky to make public appeals for a donor for their infant son, who was dying of a liver condition. A donor was found two months later, but it was too late; the baby was too sick to survive even with the new liver. Other parents have sought widespread publicity in similar situations. But injustice may occur as a result. A child who has gained much public support might, as a result of the pressure, be moved up on the list of candidates ahead of other equally needy children whose plights are largely unknown. An international society of transplant doctors has urged that measures be devised to prevent any such unfairness. It has also set guidelines designed to prevent sales of organs and to protect living kidney donors, ensuring that no pressure of any kind is put on them to make them offer to donate.

Canadian and American transplant centers have developed a system by which to share information about patients most urgently in need and to exchange organs, should hearts or kidneys become available in one country that don't match patients there but could be used in the other country. Canada has a nation-wide system through which organs are first offered to centers in Canada. About half of the organs used in transplants in Ontario come from the United States and, in turn, many American patients receive transplants from Canadian donors. Although the improved methods of overcoming rejection have made precise tissue matching less critical, patient and donor must still be matched in blood type and size and in other major factors governing compatibility. Sometimes no patient awaiting a transplant in the same region is a good enough match.

Usually, when a heart is to be donated under such circumstances, members of the transplant team fly to the hospital where a brain dead donor's heart is kept alive by machines until the transplant doctors arrive to remove it. The heart is kept cooled on the return trip to prevent tissue damage and is transplanted as soon as possible. Four or five hours, however, is about the longest a cooled heart can be preserved. Livers can last for six to eight hours and kidneys for two or three days. Until recently, lungs could not be transported outside of the body because they became damaged within an hour. But Toronto doctors have now successfully air-lifted lungs from other Ontario centers, and doctors in Pittsburgh have developed a device that allows a heart and lungs to be protected for up to eight hours. The device, a heated plexiglass box, keeps the heart pumping blood through the lungs, while air is supplied to the lungs with an inflatable bag compressed four times a minute, as if the lungs were still in a breathing person.

With an increasing number of people on waiting lists for heart–lung transplants, the new method will help some of them get transplants sooner, and help ensure that lungs potentially available for transplants do not go to waste.

Bone Marrow Transplants

In the 1960s, doctors came up with an idea that seemed incredible. Wasn't it possible, they asked, to give a whole, healthy immune system to children born lacking one, and to cure leukemia by replacing a patient's malignant white cells with healthy new ones? By that time, doctors knew that all blood cells originated in the bone marrow and that the process began with one common kind of forefather called a stem cell. They could move healthy stem cells from one person to another by means of a bone marrow transplant. The idea proved sound, but as they discovered over the next 20 years, the road to success was a bumpy one.

The catch was that by extracting marrow from the large bones of a donor and injecting it into a patient, they were putting into the patient the very cells that attack foreign tissue. The immune cells, produced by the transplanted bone marrow, would view the patient as foreign. The patient's "self" antigens (which doctors call human leukocyte antigens) would not look like self at all to the donor's cells, and they would be attacked by cells from the transplant. Doctors call the phenomenon graft versus host disease (GVHD).

At first, the only bone marrow transplants performed were in patients who had a healthy identical twin. Identical twins begin as a single fertilized egg and so have the same genes. Genes carry the code for everything that makes up the body, including human leukocyte antigens, so each twin is considered as self by the other's T cells, and GVHD doesn't occur.

But, of course, the number of such patients was very limited. As scientists learned more about the genes governing self antigens, they were able to determine whether or not two children with the same parents had inherited the same kinds of self antigen genes or at least some that matched. Two children in a family may both inherit some similar self genes, just as they can each inherit blue eyes or daddy's big nose. There is a one in four chance that such children will match in genes governing the most important self antigens. Each person inherits half of his or her genetic material from each parent.

Tests were developed that could tell when the tissue of

two siblings was compatible. Bone marrow transplants were extended to patients who had matched donors in the family. About four in every 10 persons whose lives might be saved by bone marrow transplant have a brother or sister who matches. But there was a wrinkle. Scientists could identify the major self antigens, and therefore predict reasonably well when a sibling would be a suitable donor. But T cells, which are the white cells that recognize self from non-self, can detect subtle differences, too. Some 60 per cent of patients with matched donors developed GVHD despite the match.

As in other kinds of transplants, there was also the possibility that the patient's immune cells would cause rejection by attacking the transplant cells. That wasn't a problem for children born with combined immune deficiency. Children lacking immune systems of their own couldn't reject the transplant; they were bereft of the immune cells that would attack foreign tissue. But as bone marrow transplants were given for other reasons — for instance to patients with leukemia or severe life-threatening anemia from a shortage of red blood cells — ways had to be found to prevent the patient's defense mechanism from destroying the donor bone marrow. In any case, in leukemia patients it is necessary to get rid of all cancerous white cells. Radiation or drugs or both are used to eliminate the patient's own white cells, to prevent rejection and to make room in the blood for a new population of healthy cells that will develop from the donor marrow.

In recent years, scientists have found that they can control graft versus host disease by taking T cells out of the donor marrow before it is given the patient. Different methods have been devised. One involves making antibodies in the laboratory to the donor T cells, hooking the antibodies to a toxic material, ricin (made from castor beans), and then treating the bone marrow with the antibodies. The antibodies attach themselves to antigens on the T cells and the ricin kills the T cells. Another method uses a soy bean product that, like a magnet, attracts T cells and causes them to clump so they can be removed.

Preventing graft versus host disease by such techniques has meant that bone marrow transplants today work exceedingly well in children with combined immune deficiency, proving successful in more than 90 per cent of cases. They are also effective in children with an inherited condition called Wiscott-Aldrich syndrome, which is believed to be a macrophage deficit that causes poor, although not total absence of, body defenses.

But the immune system had an unpleasant surprise for doctors. In Seattle, Dr. Donnall Thomas, one of the pioneers of bone marrow transplants, discovered that in some patients given marrow from which T cells have been removed, the transplant fails to work. It was a shock, he said, because he and his co-workers had become accustomed to having every single transplant "take" successfully. No one knows why removing T cells may interfere with a patient's ability to accept a transplant. Dr. Thomas also found that children with one kind of leukemia in whom a graft versus host disease was prevented did not do as well as those who suffered from GVHD. Their leukemia returned. It is possible that the same cells that cause GHVD — certain T cells from the donor — may also attack cancer cells. Dr. Thomas has suggested that T cells in the transplant may help stop a recurrence of the cancer by destroying any new leukemia cells that turn up. There is as yet, however, no proven explanation.

Nevertheless, being able to remove T cells from marrow has made it possible for bone marrow transplants to be given successfully to people for whom there are no ideally matched donors. While partially matched relatives have been the donors in most cases, donors need not be related at all; like blood donors, bone marrow donors could come from the general population. Volunteers would not give marrow, however, until it was needed for a particular patient. Their names would be kept on a list, along with information about their tissue typing, and they would be called on when a good match to a patient was indicated. Such volunteer lists are being compiled in England and the U.S., and a pilot project has been conducted in Canada in the Ottawa region.

Many genetic diseases affecting blood can be cured by a bone marrow transplant, because this can give a patient a new supply of healthy blood cells of all sorts to fill in for those missing in their own systems. One example is thalassemia, a condition in which red blood cells are too rapidly destroyed, causing anemia. Children born with severe types of the condition require repeated blood transfusions. Sometimes such inherited conditions are life-threatening.

Because of the potential complications that can occur, bone marrow transplants are used only when patients are at risk of dying. But by 1985, more than 200 children with genetic diseases who had received successful marrow transplants were living quite normal lives. More than 30 kinds of genetic diseases have been reported to be successfully treated.

Doctors says genetic engineering may one day make cures for all sorts of genetic diseases possible. Then doctors will be able to help people make healthy blood cells of their own. But that can't be done yet; for the time being, the next best therapy for such patients is a transplant that will generate an on-going supply of another person's blood cells in place of their own. Without an understanding of the immune system, it wouldn't have been possible to recreate a healthy blood-forming system in a person whose life was at stake. Today, in many medical centers, bone marrow transplants bring triumph over death.

Blood Transfusions

Every year in North America, about five million blood transfusions are given. Millions of us donate blood and many of us, at some time in our lives, may need blood. Blood transfusions are as familiar as traffic lights. When we learned that AIDS could be spread in transfused blood, it was alarming. It threw open to doubt and worry the safety of a transfusion should we need one.

For centuries, blood transfusions were unsafe, but it had nothing to do with AIDS. In the 17th century, attempts were made to transfuse blood. But it was not until the 19th century that anyone had any idea why it was that a transfusion sometimes caused no trouble at all and at other times could make a patient desperately ill or even cause death. The reason, as the scientist Karl Landsteiner discovered at the turn of the century, was that some people had certain antigens on their red blood cells while others did not. Today, we know those antigens as A and B. A person who does not have them is said to have Type O blood. A person with only A has type A blood, or with only B, type B blood. A small percentage of people have both A and B, and thus are type AB.

Type O is the most common. For every eight people

with Type O blood in North America, there are seven with Type A, two with type B and one with AB. Your blood type is inherited. If you are Type A, for example, you have always had the A antigen and so your immune system recognizes it as part of you and does not attack it. However, if your blood was given to a Type O person, antibodies to that A antigen would be produced. A severe immune reaction could follow, as powerful and potentially destructive to the patient as an earthquake to a country. The Type O person's immune cells could seek to destroy all the red cells in the transfused blood. The same thing would happen in a Type B person who was given Type A blood. In his blood, the type B antigen is a natural part of red cells but the A antigen is not.

However, in most cases, a Type A or Type B person can safely be given Type O blood, since it has no native antigens that would trigger an immune response. Nevertheless, because the Type O person could have been exposed to antigens A or B some time before and have produced antibodies to them, it is safer to give matched blood transfusions, that is, to give only Type A blood to a Type A person, and so on. Antibodies to A in a transfusion of a Type O donor's blood could, when given to a Type A, cause some reaction, although it would not be nearly as severe as instances in which the antibodies belong in the patient — in such a case, the patient's immune system sees the transfusion as a massive infection.

To find out which blood type you are, technicians mix a small number of your red cells with serum containing one or the other kind of antibodies. If there is the kind of antigen on your cells that fits those antibodies, the red cells will clump together, a process doctors call agglutination. If antibodies against the A antigen caused clumping in the sample in the test tube, you would have Type A blood. As long as transfusions match the patients' A, B, or O blood type, no problem will arise, in nine cases out of 10. Those are the crucial matching markers. Blood plasma, the watery, amber fluid in blood that does not contain cells, can be given without fear of a severe transfusion reaction and has been used in extreme situations, such as wartime, when there are many casualties and there isn't time to cross-match blood for transfusions. It is the cells that carry antigens that can trigger the immune response.

But over the years, researchers have found that other

lesser antigens sometimes give trouble, too. They are the reasons people can have a reaction even when they are given blood matched for A, B, or O. In the 1940s, Dr. Landsteiner discovered antigens called Rh. The Rh name comes from the Rhesus monkey, in which they were first identified. A person who has this antigen is termed Rh positive. A lack of it is called Rh negative. It was learned that this antigen can cause the bizarre death of an unborn baby, whose red blood cells are destroyed by the mother's immune system. Such deaths, which can now be prevented, used to occur when the mother did not have the antigen (Rh negative), but the baby did, inheriting it from the father. The antibodies made against the Rh antigen are primarily IgG, the kind that can cross the placenta from the mother into the baby. Typically, the first-born child of an Rh negative mother is all right. Little antigen from the child reaches the mother during the pregnancy and so the mother has not produced a big supply of antibodies against it. At the time of birth, however, the mother comes in contact with a lot of the baby's Rh antigen. From then on, antibodies against it will be in her body. As we learned earlier, the immune system remembers from experience. If the antigen is encountered again, the immune system is ready to react swiftly and strongly, just as it would against a virus antigen.

So if the mother becomes pregnant again and the second baby has the antigen, the mother's antibodies could cause fatal red cell destruction in the baby. The rescue for such a child, if it survived to birth, was either blood transfusions to provide it with red cells, or plasma exchange, to change all the blood fluids in its body, giving the baby plasma that did not contain the lethal antibodies. Later it became possible to give a baby a transfusion before it was born. That allowed rescue of infants who were becoming too sick to survive the full pregnancy. Using monitoring techniques to determine which infants were in trouble long before they were due to be born, doctors could give an infant still in the womb blood transfusions or even total plasma exchange.

During the 1960s and 70s, major advances were made in preventing the tragedy, with the University of Manitoba in Canada leading the way in much of the research. In that province, in 1963 and 1964, there were 55 such baby deaths, but 10 years later only one death occurred in a two-year period. The first step forward was the discovery of a way to prevent Rh negative women from making the dangerous antibodies. Here's how it works: an immunoglobulin, a preparation made of antibodies against the unwanted, lethal antibodies, is injected into an Rh negative woman, pregnant for the first time, as soon as her baby is born. For many such women, that is soon enough to stop the formation of antibodies. Since 1975, however, the immunoglobulin has been given even sooner, at the 28th week of pregnancy. Today, very few women ever develop the antibodies and those who had already developed them before there was immunoglobulin for prevention are, for the most part, getting past child-bearing years. Doctors predict that in the western world, the death of a baby for this reason will be a rare event indeed. An understanding of the immune system has virtually wiped out a heart-breaking baby killer.

Oddly enough, while A, B, and O matching is essential in blood transfusions, a mother and her baby can be a mismatch in those antigens with no trouble caused to the baby. It is quite different from the Rh antigen. Antibodies to A and B antigens are chiefly IgM, a class of antibody that can't cross the placenta from mother to child.

Other antibodies may also be involved in transfusion reactions. They are not as important, ordinarily, as blood type antibodies. However, people who have had a number of transfusions, or women who have been pregnant more than once, may have had earlier encounters with lesser red cell antigens that will bring forth a strong response if they are encountered again. The earlier encounters may have been so long beforehand that antibodies are at levels too low to detect in tests used to match blood; the immune system, however, like an elephant, never forgets. Some memory cells that know of a past encounter are still around. Within 72 hours to several days after the new exposure, the immune system will be on the attack. The reaction may show up as mild jaundice.

A different reason for a reaction stems from the fact that many people don't produce IgA. Most of them would never be aware of it — although they might wonder why they had more than their share of respiratory illnesses — until they needed a blood transfusion. Should they be given blood that contained IgA, they could well make antibodies against it and suffer possibly even a severe reaction. A study by the

Canadian Red Cross found that among 21 people who lacked IgA and had reactions, 12 had created antibodies against IgA that they had received in transfusions. Screening the blood of more than 200,000 healthy donors, the Red Cross found about one in 500 lacked IgA. Some studies have indicated that people lacking IgA are more prone to auto-immune diseases such as arthritis or thyroid disease. Just why that may be so has not been explained.

Until AIDS came along, the disease spread in transfused blood that most worried physicians was hepatitis. It is still a problem. Since 1971, however, a test to screen blood for hepatitis B virus particles in blood has reduced the risk enormously. The test is not 100 per cent foolproof but is nearly so. But there is no widely used screening test for another kind of hepatitis, called non A–non B. The symptoms are usually mild but an estimated one-third of people who get it develop chronic hepatitis.

While the risk of getting this kind of hepatitis from blood is far greater than the risk of getting AIDS, the potential deadliness of AIDS makes it more frightening. Some people have been so fearful that they have wanted to provide their own blood donors if they are undergoing surgery and may need blood. Usually hospitals are unwilling to allow patients to make these private arrangements; if many patients made such requests, the blood banks couldn't keep up with the extra work involved. Since 1985, donated blood in Canada and the U.S. has been screened for AIDS with a test that detects antibodies to the AIDS virus. Antibodies demonstrate that the person has had contact at some time with the virus. But they do not mean every person with antibodies will get AIDS.

In the first two months that blood in Canada was screened, 45 samples among 182,000 blood donations contained the antibodies. Such blood is not used for transfusions but may be studied at laboratories conducting AIDS research. The rate in Canada — 25 per 100,000 donations — is lower than the U.S. rate, which is 38 per 100,000 donations. Blood is screened first with a rapid test; samples that are positive for antibodies are taken through a more complex test to rule out false positives.

Both Canadian and American Red Cross doctors have repeatedly stressed that the blood transfusion supply is safe.

Many doctors, nevertheless, will feel more certain about reassuring their patients not to worry if it becomes possible to screen blood not just for antibodies but also for the virus itself. At the moment, a person could carry the virus but have caught it too recently for antibodies to have formed. Some studies in the U.S. have disclosed that about a quarter of people carrying the virus don't make antibodies for several months. Thus it is likely a handful of infected blood donations will slip through the screen. But blood products made from them are heat-treated today and have proven safe. The AIDS virus is sensitive to heat and unable to cause infection after being subjected to high temperature. But even with safe blood as a result of screening, we will, for the next few years, hear of people infected by transfusions they received before screening began. The AIDS virus can remain silent in the body for up to five years before it causes illness.

In Canada, those people found by the Canadian Red Cross blood service to have AIDS antibodies are asked, by letter, to supply the name of their family doctor. The doctor is notified and expected to advise the patient on what the test means. Such people are asked not to give blood or donate organs for transplant or sperm for artificial insemination. Men are urged to use condoms during sexual intercourse. Women are cautioned not to get pregnant, because the virus can be passed from mother to unborn child.

In the United States, hospitals are undertaking the huge task of identifying patients who were given, in the past, transfusions of blood from people who now have AIDS antibodies. Physicians of those patients are notified. They are required to inform their patients that they might have been exposed to the virus at the time of the transfusion; the donor might have been infected before screening tests were available.

Researchers are delving into the field of blood substitutes. Some day, artificial blood made of substances that can transport oxygen, but that carry none of the risks of infection or reaction of human blood, may be widely available. So far the products produced are of limited use, but progress is being made in improving them.

Surgery can be performed without the need for blood transfusions. Even major surgery, such as open heart surgery, has been done on patients who refuse blood transfusions, such as Jehovah's Witnesses, who object on religious grounds.

Some surgeons recommend that the blood a patient loses during surgery be collected in the operating room and returned to the patient. Machines that suction up blood and filter it efficiently make the procedure safe, the doctors say. There is no question that the safest transfusion of all is a transfusion of your own blood. But even if many surgeons adopted the blood recycling measures, there will remain a need for transfusions or blood products for accident victims who suffer substantial blood loss, for people with hemophilia (bleeders' disease), and for other people whose own blood supply is not good enough.

Doctors have discovered one group of patients for whom blood transfusions have a beneficial side-effect. People undergoing kidney transplants are less likely to reject the organ if they have had blood transfusions. At one time, doctors thought that the reason for this was that blood transfusions cause suppression of the immune system. But more recent findings indicate that the opposite is true: The immune system is revved up by antigens in the transfusions, and immune cells are activated and reproduce themselves. While they are reproducing, they are more vulnerable to the immune-suppressant drugs that are given kidney transplant patients. In effect, rejection appears to be prevented because more of the cells that might attack the new kidney are destroyed.

In both transplants and transfusions, it often seems that the mechanisms that are intended to protect a person work against the new organ or blood that would save his or her life. Nature, obviously, had not anticipated that mankind would one day be so generous as to give the greatest gift possible — a part of one's own body — to save the life of another. Yet, as is often the case, the giver receives. Because of transplants, the enigma of the immune system is unfolding before our eyes, revealing new ways to rid man of much disease and suffering, once the lot of so many. From mankind's gift, a godsend for mankind.

CHAPTER 8

Cancer: Marshalling Body Defenses Against Tumors

At a cancer research meeting recently, one eminent scientist exclaimed, "This is the most exciting time in the 25 years I've been working in cancer." There was no disagreement from the audience, because doctors are on the threshold of having at their command a new approach to cancer treatment. Studies of the immune system are teaching doctors how the body's own defense system may combat malignancy. Eventually, scientists will know how to help immune cells win. In coming years we will be hearing of any number of substances that scientists have obtained from the immune system and are testing against cancer. We can expect to have our hopes raised sky-high and, sad to say, dashed again — more than once — before enough is known about the

139

intricate immune mechanisms for doctors to manipulate them successfully. We have already seen the tip of the iceberg: interferon, tumor necrosis factor (a puzzling two-edged sword to be described later in this chapter), interleukin-2, and antibodies made in the laboratory. They are not the absolute cure for cancer that we long for, but they prove that treatment via the immune system, called immunotherapy, is possible.

For many years, scientists have said that the immune system is the key to the puzzle of cancer. They believed it must know how to search out malignant cells and destroy them. Doctors could see that people with deficient immune systems were at higher risk of developing cancer, and the same held true in patients whose immune cells were deliberately held in check by drugs to prevent rejection of a transplanted organ. Other patients treated for cancer with drugs that inadvertently suppressed the body defense mechanism were sometimes cured of their initial cancer only to be confronted a few years later with the tragic irony of a second cancer, often leukemia, as the price to be paid for the cure.

In the past few years, the newly identified deadly disease AIDS, which wipes out immune cell protection, has demonstrated clearly how readily cancer can occur when the body's guardians are destroyed. Among the first 5,000 AIDS patients in the United States, 30 per cent developed a kind of cancer called Kaposi's sarcoma. Beforehand, that kind of cancer had been seen in some transplant patients, but rarely. Ordinarily it occurred only in elderly Eastern European men, who were believed to be genetically prone to it. The older men, however, got a less severe form, usually only showing up as purple skin blotches, while AIDS patients developed a more deadly form, affecting internal organs.

A number of doctors have suggested that we all have cells that turn malignant during our lifetime and that it probably happens frequently. But those cells are quickly spotted and killed. We don't all get cancer. Yet, one in four of us does, and certainly the majority of cancer patients have not taken immune-suppressant drugs nor have they had diseases that ruin their body defenses. Why didn't their immune systems rid the body of tumor cells? On the other hand, when immune cells do attack and kill cancer cells, what told them that those cells were sick?

The answers to these two questions have proved uncommonly difficult to find. One would think cancer cells should be easy for immune cells to identify. If you look at a tumor under the microscope, you may see quite clear differences between tumor cells and normal cells. Cancer cells often look weird — peculiarly shaped and too big — and, furthermore, they pile up on each other in higgledy-piggledy fashion. Normal cells are uniform in shape and orderly. Yet cancer cells may not be identified as enemies. "Somehow cancer cells manage to present a friendly face and evade body defense mechanisms," says one Canadian cancer specialist. The "face," he says, is made up of molecules that give a cell its identity. Other cells recognize these molecules, just as you recognize the faces of your neighbors and know they belong on your street. If one of your neighbors became a criminal, you might not know it from his looks. A malignant cell, unrecognized by immune warriors, may conceal its criminal intentions, too.

Nevertheless, doctors figured there must be something, some marker, on a tumor cell that gives away its true identity. Otherwise the immune system would never detect malignant cells and we'd all develop cancer. A quarter of a century ago, scientists in England and the United States proved that at least some tumor cells trigger an immune response. Since then, hundreds of cancer researchers have searched for molecules on or in cancer cells that would mark them as different from other cells. They call these elusive markers "tumor antigens." (Antigen is the name given to any molecule the immune system recognizes; it can be like a red flag to a bull.)

But the search for tumor antigens has proved incredibly frustrating. So far, scientists simply cannot find antigens that are exclusive to tumor cells, though they have isolated some antigens on tumor cells found only rarely on other cells. One of the first of these was called carcino-embryonic antigen (CEA), first identified in Montreal by McGill University scientists Dr. Phil Gold and Dr. Sam Freedman. CEA can be detected in the blood of patients with digestive tract cancers and some other kinds of diseases. The antigens are not found in healthy adults. They can be located, however, in unborn babies (embryos) early in pregnancy. CEA is widely used in the diagnosis of certain cancers and in determining the effectiveness of treatment. Levels of CEA in the blood fall, when treatment is successful, but rise again if the cancer comes back.

In the past several years, researchers have had a new, exquisitely sensitive tool with which to search for tumor antigens. Its discovery won the Nobel prize in 1984 for Dr. Georges Koehler and Dr. Cesar Milstein of Cambridge, England. Called a hybridoma (a hybrid cell formed of fusing two cells), it is a method of producing in the laboratory a supply of specific antibodies. It is like having a tame B cell that puts out an endless stream of identical antibodies. Scientists call them monoclonal antibodies. The technique has opened the door wide to new methods of diagnosis and treatment of cancer. It lets doctors make specific antibodies against molecules of tumor cells. The antibodies will then track down and attach themselves to other cells bearing those same molecules. Most, if not all, of the other cells will also be tumor cells.

Now scientists have found ways to attach radioactive material that shows up under a scanning machine to such antibodies. Doctors can see the radioactive material and thus know where the antibodies are in the body. With the scanning machine, they show up as dots of light. The cells the antibodies have attached themselves to are most likely tumor cells; doctors can observe if the cancer has spread. Drugs can also be hooked to the antibodies and be transported directly to tumor cells, poisoning those cells without affecting nearby healthy cells.

Cancer doctors have always dreamed of a "magic bullet" that would shoot down tumor cells but not other cells. Monoclonal antibodies may make that dream come true, and countless experiments are under way to devise such treatments. Some patients have already been treated, with encouraging results.

In Britain, doctors have been able to detect cancer spreading to bone marrow in women with breast cancer by using monoclonal antibodies against tumor-related antigens; the antibodies tracked down cancer cells spreading to bone much earlier than such microscopic new nests of cancer cells could be found by any other method. From a group of these women, doctors removed a portion of bone marrow and treated it with antibodies hooked to a plant toxin, abrin, to get rid of any tumor cells. Meantime, the patients were given drugs to destroy the rest of the bone marrow still in their bodies; it might still harbor cancer cells. Their own cleansed bone marrow was returned. It will replace bone marrow that was removed. In effect, they were given bone marrow transplants of their own marrow, once it had been scoured of tumor cells. The same technique has been used in patients with blood cell cancers in the United States; their sick blood cells were destroyed and the clean bone marrow produced healthy blood cells.

A number of other studies are under way. In British Columbia, scientists have found a way to hook tumor-associated antibodies to a molecule called porphyrin, a natural substance found in plant chlorophyll. Exposed to light, porphyrin reacts violently, firing oxygen molecules that blow holes in cell walls. In animal experiments, injected antibody–porphyrin particles were set off by controlled doses of light. Tumors in half of the animals were eliminated. In Texas, scientists have begun treating leukemia patients with antibodies attached to a plant poison, ricin. A British scientist, working with researchers in California, is testing plant toxins and cancer drugs hooked to antibodies to treat colon cancer. Montreal scientists are using antibodies to seek out a protein called oncomodulin. Commonly found in some kinds of cancer, this protein provides a diagnostic test. And in Philadelphia, doctors have attached macrophages to the antibodies. The macrophages, towed to the tumor site, attack cancer cells. Some 300 patients have undergone the treatment and about half have benefited. They had tumors of bowel, pancreas, and stomach. A few have been free of disease for more than three years.

While making use of antibodies to zero in on cancer cells is a promising new way to get at tumor cells that have spread (metastasis), it isn't expected that antibodies *per se* will prove to be powerful cancer cell killers. In the body, antibodies are not known to fight cancer effectively. Indeed, certain antibodies can hide tumor cells from T cells, in the same way they hide an unborn baby from attack by the mother's immune cells. They cover up the molecules that the T cells might see were not normal bits of the body. Like a fetus, tumor cells appear able to coat themselves with protective antibodies, and also to send out signals to suppress an attack by destructive antibodies. One of the chemical signals is called alphafetoprotein, which lowers the potency of an immune response. Like CEA, it is found in some adults with tumors, and in fetuses.

Scientists would dearly love to know how to turn on the immune system to make it recognize and kill cancer cells. As long ago as the late 19th century, New York physician Dr. William B. Coley noted that tumors in his patients sometimes shrank when they got a bacterial infection. He began treating patients with a mixture of killed bacteria that caused their immune systems to react as if they had a real infection. The material was called Coley's toxin; sometimes it worked, sometimes it didn't. In 1916, he reported successful treatment of eight out of 29 patients with malignant melanoma — cancer of skin pigment cells — the most dangerous form of skin cancer. But, for the most part, the medical establishment considered the treatment as verging on quackery. For three-quarters of a century it was ignored. Other scientists had tried, with some success, injecting another substance that can arouse the immune system. Known as BCG (bacille Calmette-Guerin), it is used in a vaccine against tuberculosis. Although some reports of good results were published, most studies found that the therapy was not impressive. The idea had been put on the shelf.

But in 1975, at Memorial Sloan-Kettering Cancer Center in New York, Dr. Lloyd Old and colleagues once again looked at Dr. Coley's theory. They injected into mice with tumors a substance called endotoxin that was extracted from the cells walls of certain strains of bacteria. The tumors turned black and died. Doctors call such tissue death necrosis. The endotoxin did not kill the tumor cells, but a substance the mice themselves produced as a result of the endotoxin injection did. Dr. Old found this substance in blood stream of the mice.

The scientists gave the substance the name of tumor necrosis factor (TNF). When researchers collected blood serum from mice treated with TNF and mixed it with cancer cells in a culture dish, the cancer cells died. Normal cells, however, did not. The researchers also re-examined BCG and found that it causes macrophages to multiply rapidly. When they gave the mice both BCG and TNF, levels of TNF in mouse serum rose substantially, indicating that macrophages are likely the cells that produce TNF. Since then, it has been discovered that macrophages in humans also produce TNF. In 1983, Dr. Old determined that TNF was most effective against tumor cells when it was mixed with interferon. Interferon is also a substance produced by immune cells.

But for TNF researchers a dismaying pitfall lay ahead: TNF turned out to be identical to the substance produced in the body that makes cancer patients waste away. (We'll come to that part of the story in a moment.)

To the scientific world, the discovery of natural anti-tumor agents, such as TNF and interferon, has been electrifying. At last, scientists had available to them products that the immune system uses when it doctors the body. Other chemicals made by immune cells, including interleukins, were under intense study. The immune system had seemed, previously, to be a baffling black box; now its lid had been pried open a crack.

The public, however, was disillusioned. Interferon first burst onto the scene in the 1970s. Despite the cautions of many cancer doctors who warned us that interferon research would be slow going, people believed it was going to work wonders for cancer patients immediately. They were badly disappointed; it performed no instant miracles. (We'll come back to interferon a little later.)

Tumor necrosis factor (TNF) received less hype in the general news media. But in the pharmaceutical industry in the United States, Europe, and Japan, TNF set off high hopes for a winning product and a race to produce the material in the laboratory by means of genetic engineering. An American company achieved it in 1984, and by 1985 a Japanese company had its version ready to be tested in 100 desperately ill patients.

But at Rockefeller University in New York — just across the street from Memorial Sloan-Kettering, where tumor necrosis factor was discovered — and at the Weizmann Institute of Science in Israel, scientists were studying a protein, cachectin, that caused severe weight loss and debilitation in people with certain severe infections and in about one-third of cancer patients. Fortuitously, the Rochester scientists sent a sample of cachectin to a researcher in California at the Scripps Clinic and Research Foundation where tumor necrosis factor was under study. Scripps personnel compared the molecular make-up of the two substances and were startled by the results; the two proteins were the same. The Israeli scientists also reported the match.

Now scientists believe that in low doses the protein, produced by macrophages, fights malignancy; high doses, however, initiate changes in fat metabolism that lead to wasting. They suspect the reason for the change in metabolism is to move fat out of storage so it can be used elsewhere during the battle against disease. But beyond a certain point, that strategy boomerangs; patients become so debilitated that life is threatened or lost. In small groups of patients tested with tumor necrosis factor, no improvement was seen. As more is learned, TNF may find its niche in cancer therapy. So far, the risk appears to outweigh the benefit.

Yet another exhilarating development came late in 1985. At the U.S. National Cancer Institute, Dr. Steven Rosenberg (President Ronald Reagan's cancer surgeon) and colleagues reported treating 25 patients with a new therapy involving interleukin-2, a substance made by T cells. They had found that taking white cells from a patient and giving the cells interleukin-2 could turn certain cells into super killers of tumor cells. They could watch them destroying the cancer cells in laboratory dishes. The cells were then returned to the patient along with more interleukin-2. Eleven of the 25 patients improved. One 29-year-old woman was freed of malignant melanoma that had spread all over her body; the tumors of 10 others shrank to half the former size or less. The cells that became fierce killers were null cells, lymphocytes in the blood that are neither T cells nor B cells and about which not a great deal is known.

When the report was made public, telephone lines at the institute were jammed with calls. Thousands of people phoned, pleading for the treatment for themselves or their loved ones. "It was heart-rending," an institute spokesman said later. There was no way the treatment could be given to large numbers of people at that time, even if doctors had been much surer than they were of its effectiveness. But doctors don't even know yet how safe the treatment is, much less whether it will live up to its early promise. Of the first 49 patients treated, 18 benefited; their tumors shrank. It will be some years before it becomes widely available, should results continue to look encouraging as more people receive it. The treatment is not without hazards; it can cause fluid retention leading to breathing difficulties. One patient died from this complication and two others had severe respiratory problems. Furthermore, nobody yet knows how long the patients who improved will remain better. The treatment is too new for any predictions.

The institute can only treat eight patients at a time. For two weeks, Monday to Friday, they are hooked up to a machine to have lymphocytes collected from their blood, four hours each day. The cells are then cultured for three or four days with interleukin-2. Null cells that have become killers are extracted from the culture. These cells have been named lymphokine activated killer cells or LAK cells. The LAK cells are reinfused into the patient's vein, and interleukin-2 is administered every eight hours. Most patients had the two-week cycle of treatment repeated. It involves a long stay in hospital and costs thousands of dollars. If it can save lives, the side-effects and costs may be a price worth paying. Dr. Rosenberg has said it may be possible to prevent some adverse effects and to make the therapy less complex and less costly. But it is still a big if, as he is the first to admit. Doctors at some other American medical centers have begun testing the method. In Canada and other countries, where studies of interleukin-2 have been progressing for some time, scientists had observed that it killed tumors in mice and human tumor cells grown in the laboratory. They have discovered that two or three kinds of killer cells become active when they receive interleukin-2. Dr. Rosenberg's patients included people with lung, kidney, rectal, and colon cancers, and in many the disease had spread to other sites. In most cases, it was the secondary tumors that shrank with the treatment. This is significant because it is the spread of cancer that makes the disease deadly. Describing the treatment, Dr. Rosenberg said: "This is really the first step. It demonstrates that it is possible to manipulate the immune system and make a variety of cancers in a variety of locations disappear."

At Harvard Medical School, doctors are trying a different version of Dr. Rosenberg's treatment. Instead of harvesting cells from the blood to turn them into killers, they collect lymphocytes attached to the tumor and give them a booster with interleukin-2. The doctors think these specific white cells already recognize the tumor cells as enemies; the booster increases their numbers.

Interleukin-2 was discovered in 1976 by the co-discoverer of the AIDS virus, Dr. Robert Gallo of the U.S. National Cancer Institute. Scientists have learned how to produce it in the laboratory, making it plentiful enough for study and tests. They have discovered receptors that cells create to catch interleukin-2. Those receptors appear on the outer coats of cells when the cell becomes active. Normally they are not present when a cell is resting. But researchers have found large numbers of such receptors on some leukemic cells — particularly T cells that have been turned malignant by a cancer virus called HTLV-I. This cancer is rare in North America, but common in parts of Japan and the Caribbean. The finding has led to a new approach to treatment, using monoclonal antibodies against the receptors. The aim is to stop T cells from proliferating wildly (leukemia is abnormal growth of white cells). In early tests, patients had temporary remissions (freedom from symptoms) of their disease. Without receptors to take in interleukin-2, necessary for cell reproduction, the sick T cells could not multiply.

A spin-off from this cancer research may be a new treatment for auto-immune diseases, such as diabetes, in which T cells attack normal parts of the body. Interfering with the transmission of interleukin-2 with the drug cyclosporine A looks promising, leading researchers to try antibodies as another method of jamming the interleukin-2 signal. (See Chapter Three, on auto-immune diseases.) If antibodies work as an alternate method of interfering, they might prove less toxic than drugs.

We begin to grasp the complexity of our immune systems when we see that sometimes adding a cell product such as interleukin-2, and sometimes blocking the substance out, helps fight cancer. Understanding what our defense cells do and the substances they produce arises from studies called basic research. Basic research isn't aimed specifically at devising treatments or cures for disease; therefore, we often find it difficult to recognize its importance. Currently, a great deal of cancer research involves work being done by basic researchers: cell biologists, molecular biologists, and genetic scientists. Many of us have scanty understanding of the microscopic world in which they make their discoveries, and we sometimes feel little progress is being made in cancer research. Our pessimism is not justified. Today's discoveries of mechanisms underlying our body defenses will provide the basis for effective therapies in future. But it's hard to be patient. Why can't they harness the immune system more quickly?

The problem doctors face when they attempt to use substances made by the immune system to treat patients is many-sided. There is little question that these substances are extremely powerful. The body makes them in tiny amounts and doesn't keep them around for long. They are bound to be toxic and have adverse effects. It will take a long time to learn how to use them. Immune cells make many different substances, and little is known about how these substances interact with each other to keep the system in balance. It isn't even known how many products immune cells make; there may be hundreds of them remaining to be discovered. Much mystery cloaks the actions of those that have been detected.

Researchers have already suggested that immune system products might have to be doled out in cocktails containing more than one substance. Learning how to use them in combinations will take time. Consider how long it is taking to gain an understanding of interferon.

Interferon has demonstrated only modest success in a limited number of cancers when it is used alone. Known to exist for many years, it has been studied intensely since 1980, but it still produces surprises, nudging doctors to remind them that they don't know everything about interferon yet. Among one group of patients who had been treated with interferon for a few months, for example, two grew extraordinarily long eyelashes. Left untrimmed, one woman's eyelashes curled up on her forehead and down her cheeks, according to a report. By the second year of treatment, the two patients had to cut their eyelashes twice a week. Both patients had cancer of the lymphatic system, non-Hodgkin's lymphoma. The hair on their heads was not affected, but pubic hair was. Doctors could not explain why.

Interferon was discovered more than a quarter of a century ago by two scientists, one British and one Swiss. In cells attacked by a virus, one kind of interferon is produced that slows down the viruses' ability to multiply; but it could be obtained from blood in only small amounts, and a number of years passed before doctors acquired large enough quantities of interferon to study. In 1980, by means of genetic engineering, it became possible to produce interferon in the laboratory. It was still fairly expensive; a teaspoonful cost $250 to $300 dollars. Doctors have been trying it against a wide variety of cancers.

So far, the one kind of cancer it can control is a rare but deadly form of leukemia called hairy cell leukemia, because cells are surrounded by hair-like appendages. The cells collect in the spleen, enlarging the organ, and proliferate in bone marrow, replacing normal blood cells. Until interferon, no treatment was highly effective. Of more than 60 patients treated at the University of Chicago, 85 per cent achieved at least partial remissions. The patients inject one kind of interferon (alpha) under the skin three times a week.

In Baltimore, doctors created an artificial virus that stimulates the production of interferon in the body. Interferon is known to act on natural killer cells, immune cells that spontaneously attack and kill tumor cells. Early tests in patients with chronic leukemia showed the patients improved to some extent after a few weeks of treatment with the phony virus. Doctors are greatly interested in natural killer cells because they are believed to be a key force in protection against cancer. Studies with a breed of mice known as nude mice (for their lack of hair) disclosed that natural killer cells protect the animals against cancer tumors, without the help of T cells. T helper cells, you'll recall, give the orders to other immune cells. But nude mice are born without a thymus gland, the organ essential to the development of T cells: the mice have no T cells, yet they are no more at risk of cancer than ordinary mice. Scientists learned that the mice are protected by natural killer cells. Interferon may yet prove to have a role in stimulating these killers into combat.

Researchers at Stanford University in California have suggested that interforon's niche in the spectrum of treatments may be in preventing a recurrence of cancer, because it seems to be more a watchdog than a tumor killer. It has little effect against the major cancers of lung, breast, and colon . Given to patients whose disease has been brought under control by other methods, interferon might alert warrior cells to any new nest of tumor cells that is starting up.

Another intriguing substance made by white cells is

called transfer factor. At Cornell University, scientists obtain it by grinding up white cells from healthy donors. Given to patients with immune deficiencies who are afflicted with a chronic fungal infection (candidiasis), transfer factor acts almost magically to clear up the chronic infection. Now, at several medical centers, scientists have tested transfer factor taken from donors against cancer tumors. A donor whose white cells react against cells from a patient's tumor when mixed together in the laboratory — indicating that the donor has immunity to that particular tumor — is selected as the source of transfer factor to be given that patient. The immunity seems to be transferred to the patient. How it works is under investigation and the treatment is being tested experimentally.

Vaccines to protect us against cancer would be wonderful. There are some such vaccines against animal cancer — one, for example, to protect cattle against eye cancer, developed recently by Australian veterinarians. Cancers caused by viruses are relatively common in animals but rare in people. Two have been found: a leukemia virus and a lymphoma virus; both belong to the same sub-species of viruses as the AIDS virus. Scientists don't know, yet, if vaccines against these strange viruses are possible.

But other viruses play a role indirectly in cancer, among them the Epstein-Barr virus, the hepatitis B virus, and quite likely, some genital wart viruses. Vaccines against those viruses can, in a sense, be considered cancer vaccines. The Epstein-Barr virus — the cause of infectious mononucleosis in North America — is linked to two cancers in parts of Africa and Asia, Burkitt's lymphoma and nasopharyngeal carcinoma. Scientists, including Dr. M.A. Epstein of the University of Bristol, a discoverer of the virus bearing his name, are developing a vaccine that is close to being ready for tests in people. A vaccine against hepatitis B already exists and may reduce the incidence of liver cancer, the kind of malignancy to which it is linked. Most wart viruses don't cause cancer; they cause only the common warts that develop on the hands or plantar warts that grow on the soles of feet. But evidence has been accumulating that links genital wart viruses with cancer of the cervix, penis, and anal region; researchers are searching for vaccines to prevent such infections. Of the 40 types of wart virus, two have been identified by German scientists at the Cancer Center in Heidelberg as factors contributing to the development of genital cancers.

A long and twisted road remains to be traveled yet before immunotherapy becomes a standard form of treatment. But despite all the obstacles still to be overcome, science has made a start toward a fourth kind of cancer treatment to be added to surgery, drug therapy, and radiation. A new beachhead has been established in the war on cancer.

CHAPTER 9

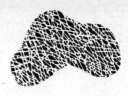

Allergies: When the Immune System Overdoes It

Are you one of a million? Every year in Canada, a million people first learn they have allergies.

It may be a group you'd rather not join. But the number of fellow sufferers is huge, greater than you may ever have realized, and is composed of people of all ages and virtually all races.

One in every six North Americans has at least one allergy. For some 40 million people, sneezes, wheezes, itches, or hives are the consequences of an encounter with something they breathe in (such as pollen or dust), or eat, or that touches their skin. For some, it is seasonal. For others, it is year round. For the lucky ones, it is only a minor inconvenience or can be prevented quite readily by avoiding the troublesome item. Yet for millions of people, allergies are a constant burden and sometimes a threat to life.

Allergic diseases that affect breathing, primarily hay fever and asthma, are the most common. About 15 per cent of the population is undergoing treatment for respiratory allergy, which tops the list of chronic illness among children and is the third most common among adults. In the United States, the 35 million Americans with allergic diseases and asthma spend more than $1-billion yearly for medical care, drugs, and hospital care.

Being allergic means that your immune system reacts to one or more substances that do not bother most people. What makes an allergy different from other ailments is that it is not caused by a harmful organism, such as a virus or bacterium. The particles that trigger an allergic reaction are, in themselves, quite innocent. They cause no reaction in most people. But in susceptible persons, the immune system mounts an attack against them wildly out of proportion to the threat. In the course of the battle, various symptoms occur: a stuffy nose, unbearably itchy eyes, hives or rashes, or an upset digestive tract causing cramps or diarrhea.

In recent years, medical scientists have begun to discover why that happens. With the new knowledge comes the possibility of exciting methods of treatment.

The word allergy dates back to 1906, coined by an Austrian physician, Baron Clemens Freiherr von Pirquet. He used it in a broader sense than we use it today; for him, allergy was any altered immune system reaction. Some years earlier, an English doctor, Charles Blackley, who like many of his patients was afflicted by hay fever with the classic symptoms of running nose and eyes, congestion, and misery, had devised what may have been the first allergy tests. He used himself as his own guinea pig. He collected pollen from dozens of plants, inhaled them, and put them under his eyelids and into his skin. He soon learned that the same pollens that brought on his hay fever symptoms also caused red, swollen patches on his skin when they were applied to scratches.

Early in the 20th century, doctors realized that something in the blood of people with allergies was causing a response to certain substances, bringing on symptoms. They called the substances that could trigger the response allergens. But it was not until 1966 that the mysterious "something in the blood" was identified. It was an antibody, identified during studies of ragweed hay fever by a husband and wife team, Kimishige and Teruko Ishizaka, at the Children's Asthma Research Institute in Denver, Colorado. This antibody, or immunoglobulin, which they named IgE, was quite different from the four kinds of antibodies already known. Compared with the others, it was produced in small amounts in normal people but in levels 10 times as high in people with allergies.

With the discovery, research took off rapidly. Before long, doctors had learned that IgE was commonly attached to cells called mast cells and basophils. Up to half a million IgE antibodies could be found on a single cell.

Mast cells are found in the skin, tongue, bladder, respiratory and digestive tracts, and connective tissue. Basophils are found in the blood. These cells cause you to sneeze in response to an allergen in an airway. They had been discovered and named in the late 1800s by Dr. Paul Erlich. In the 1930s, Swedish scientists had learned that the cells secreted heparin, a substance produced in the body to slow down the clotting of blood. Soon after that, researchers found that these cells, which are loaded with small granules, also produced histamine. Much research had already shown that histamine was somehow involved in causing symptoms of hay fever and asthma. It makes blood vessels open wider, slowing circulation and lowering blood pressure, classic symptoms of a generalized allergic response. In an allergic person, histamine seemed to appear magically when the person was exposed to an allergen. It became clear that IgE sitting on these cells had grabbed onto the allergen, signaling the cell to release powerful substances, including histamine. By 1971, scientists had been able to film the process, showing granules in a mast cell fusing with the cell's outer membrane or coat, and histamine dissolving and leaving the cell. The microscopic movie showed that the cell was left unharmed and was seemingly able to replace its granules within a few hours.

Other studies of IgE disclosed that it is produced, like the other antibodies, by B cells, one family of white cells. (See Chapter One.) The production sites are primarily the nose, tonsils, lymph nodes draining the nose, and the digestive tract. B cells producing IgE are not usually found in the spleen or lymph nodes in other parts of the body, although IgE antibodies circulate through the whole body. We all have them, but people with allergies are better at producing IgE than the rest of the population.

That might seem to be an unwanted and harmful ability. But it may have advantages, although the importance is perhaps less obvious today in developed nations than it once was. IgE is the mechanism by which the body quickly puts up a defense against a parasite invasion. It is known that IgE levels increase in people infected by parasites, such as mites that cause scabies. Hives and itching occur when the immune system combats the mites. And that makes good sense, because scratching dislodges them.

If you have an allergy to a pollen, here is the drama that takes place as you breathe in the pollen. As it gets through the nose's lining (the nasal mucosa), the pollen releases, within a couple of minutes, most of its proteins, which will set off the reaction. These proteins, which are allergens, encounter IgE antibodies sitting on mast cells. The antibodies lock onto the pollen allergens. That sends a signal into each cell to fire its weapons, histamine and other compounds. Like any other foreign particle or antigen, allergens are recognized as enemies by T cells in the area. They go into action, ordering B cells to produce antibodies, including more IgE. The T cells also send out chemical messages calling in basophil cells that have been circulating in the blood. As they arrive, the freshly produced IgE sticks to them. These IgE antibodies on the cells latch on to more allergens, so that more and more cells are sending out histamine and other compounds that make your nasal passages congested, your nose run, and your eyes stream and itch.

Your immune system is also making other kinds of antibodies, IgG and IgM; however, a person who is not allergic can breathe the same pollen but will make no detectable antibodies to the pollen at all. Much the same thing occurs in the gastrointestinal tract of people with a food allergy, although the symptoms may be abdominal cramps or diarrhea. In some cases, allergens may have spread to other tissues of the body when IgE catches up with them, so hives, or skin rashes, or eczema may occur.

Some doctors suggest that allergy to otherwise harmless inhaled particles or to certain foods may be the price one pays for having a super effective defense against parasites. It is possible that the immune system has mistaken pollen for mites, because the allergens are similar in size. According to some scientists, all known major allergens, such as ragweed, animal dander, or fish antigen, are roughly the same size. (In talking about allergies, the words allergen and antigen are synonymous. They are the molecules that the immune system recognizes and to which antibodies bind tightly.) Major allergens are those to which a majority of allergic patients respond when skin tests are done. Typically, people with allergies are allergic to a number of substances.

But knowing that nature had a reason for creating IgE, despite the fact that it often seems to be more trouble than it is worth, doesn't make allergies any easier to live with. The happy news is that research, generated by the discovery of IgE, has now uncovered more fascinating information, and doctors are getting closer to using these findings to devise better treatments. Some allergy specialists predict that cure and prevention of allergy is only five to 10 years away.

Here are some of the latest discoveries that make allergists optimistic that they are finally nearing victory. In 1982, scientists found another group of substances called leukotrienes, which, like histamine, are involved in allergies. Leukotrienes are now known to be 5,000 to 10,000 times more powerful than histamine. In people with asthma, while histamine narrows the central air passages, leukotrienes constrict the small airways of the lungs and are believed responsible for spasms of the bronchial tubes. They're also involved in inflammation in the joints of people with arthritis and are produced by cells within seconds of an injury.

Leukotrienes are produced, along with prostaglandins, another family of body chemicals, after mast cells have released their compounds on a signal from IgE. One of the compounds, in addition to histamine and heparin, released by a mast cell is arachiodonic acid, which is a component of the cell membrane. This acid, acted on by enzymes, turns into one form of leukotriene. Now scientists are finding that by blocking the production of leukotriene they can prevent asthma. At the University of California, scientists are experimenting with a unique treatment. They are replacing, through diet, arachiodonic acid with another similar fatty acid called eicosapentaenoic acid (EPA), found in cold-water fish. It does not turn into the kind of leukotriene that constricts airways or causes inflammation. But it appears that mast cells may accept EPA as a substitute for arachiodonic acid to manufacture membranes for themselves. Eskimoes have high levels of eicosapentaenoic acid because their diet is high in fish. And, interestingly, asthma is very rare in Alaskan Eskimoes. One of the California doctors says the treatment being tested on a group of severe asthmatics is "like turning them into Eskimoes." The aim of the experiment is not to devise a rigid fish diet as the answer to asthma but to learn more about preventing the unwanted effects of leukotrienes. Drugs to interfere with leukotriene production are already being studied. It seems almost certain that soon new treatments, dramatically better than today's antihistamines, will become available.

In another exciting development, researchers have found the switches that turn the production of IgE on and off. The switches are members of a family of chemicals that doctors call lymphokines, which are the language immune cells use to communicate. T cells produce two chemicals that are the switches. One is called suppressive factor of allergy; it stops production of IgE. The other, the on switch, is called enhancing factor of allergy. People with allergies may have T cells that are too quick in using the on switch or too slow in using the off switch. Studies in Japan and the U.S. that have identified the switches have helped scientists to get a handle on the problem. It could lead to ways to fine tune the production of IgE and stop it from triggering allergies.

In this scenario, suppressive factor of allergy, created in the laboratory, might be given patients at the start of an allergic attack. Or maybe T cells can be prevented from producing enhancing factor of allergy. But there is more to be learned yet. Mast cells and basophils have mechanisms by which they release histamine other than signals from IgE. Some forms of complement, the proteins in the blood that come into play when IgG and IgM antibodies latch onto antigens, can also cause the release of histamine. Allergic people produce IgG in response to allergens at the same time that they make IgE. It is complicated because some IgG antibodies can block out IgE antibodies and so help prevent allergy symptoms. Nevertheless, researchers have a firm hold on one end of the ball of yarn that is the puzzle of allergy, and steadily they are unraveling it.

It has long been said that allergies run in families. It is true that if both parents have allergies, a child is much more likely to have them. The chances range from 50 to 85 per cent. If one parent is allergic but the other is not, the chances are about 30 per cent. But the substances to which a child is allergic may not be the same allergens that affect the parents. It is the *tendency* to be allergic that is inherited, not a specific allergy to, say, ragweed or shrimp. Immune response genes are the inherited genetic material that governs that tendency, carrying instructions for the on and off switches. However, even children born to parents who don't have allergies have a one in 10 chance of developing an allergy at some time in life. Doctors have demonstrated that they can make anybody allergic, even people who have never had an allergy, if they expose them to certain doses, frequently enough to make them sensitive, of a particular allergen. The only persons who cannot develop an allergy are those whose immune systems are so defective they cannot effectively defend the body from any intruder, much less allergens.

Allergies can be a threat to life if they cause a reaction so severe the person goes into shock. Doctors call the condition anaphylaxis or allergic shock. It may start with a feeling of great uneasiness, dizziness, and nausea. The throat or airways may close up with swelling and the person feels suffocated. Blood pressure drops dramatically and the patient may collapse within a minute or two. Emergency treatment with adrenalin is crucial. It is very rare for inhaled particles to cause anaphylaxis. Sudden exposure to allergens in the form of insect stings, drugs, or food additives are more common hazards for those allergic to them. Your doctor is the best person to talk to about your risk of a severe allergic reaction. Ask the doctor to outline exactly what to do should the emergency arise. Doctors may want to prescribe for some patients, to keep in their homes or take with them on travels, a kit that contains the essential medicine to counter allergic shock.

People with allergies, possibly more than people with

any other chronic condition, need to know as much as they can about their disease. Nobody but themselves can be on guard for them day after day, to help them stay well by avoiding exposure to allergens as far as possible, or taking care of themselves when exposure can't be avoided. It has been estimated that 85 per cent of the $100-million it costs in Canada each year to treat episodes of allergic reactions is spent to treat attacks that could have been prevented.

HAY FEVER

About eight of every 10 people who consult an allergist (a doctor who specializes in treating allergies) have symptoms of hay fever, which is also called allergic rhinitis. Rhinitis means swollen nose. The term hay fever was coined 200 years ago by an English physician, John Bostock, who used it to describe his "summer cold." But mankind was suffering from hay fever long before Dr. Bostock gave it a name. The symptoms were listed by Hippocrates, the father of medicine, 2,500 years ago. Most of us have either suffered the symptoms or observed somebody with them: an itchy, stuffy, runny, nose; itchy, weeping eyes; blocked sinuses; a sore or itchy throat. Some people find the back of their throat so itchy that they reach in with a toothbrush to scratch it. Some sufferers look as if they've been partying all night. Dark circles under their eyes make them seem exhausted. Called allergic shiners, they are caused by nasal congestion obstructing blood flow in veins, so that pools of dark-coloured venous blood collect under the eyes.

Few of us are aware of it, but our noses follow a cycle. The nose is continually switching from one passage to another, with one passage open and the other closed. Smells, which stimulate scent nerve endings in the nose, make you feel as if you are breathing more clearly. That's why some cough drops, or even garlic, seem to help when you have a stuffy nose. And if your nose always seems most congested at night when you are trying to sleep, it is because when you lie down, nose tissue swells and muscles that keep the nose open relax.

People whose rhinitis is seasonal are probably allergic to plant pollen. The time of year is a tip-off to the kind of plant. In spring, the trouble-maker is most likely tree pollen. Birch trees are a particular problem in parts of Canada and in Scandinavia, but oak, maple, or elm trees may also be the source. In summer, drying grasses send pollen out on the breeze, and in autumn, weeds are awaiting their turn to make people sneeze. Ragweed is considered the major producer of allergens in North America, although not in Europe, where grasses head the list. Mugwort is another bothersome weed.

Pollen is the male part of plants. Humans are "accidental intruders in the life cycle of plants," says one allergist. A plant, in its inherent drive to reproduce, sends out billions of pollen grains. Plants that produce tiny grains put them aboard the wind, and they are the ones we breathe in. Most flowers make larger grains and use insects as transportation vehicles. The windborn male grains are in search of their female counterparts, the sticky hairs of the stigma, a plant's egg-bearing organ. Those grains carried by the wind to a mate soak up moisture from the stigma and then flush it back out, loaded with plant proteins. If the female is the same species, it too sends out answering proteins and fertilization occurs. But male pollen grains can't tell the moist, sticky surface of your nose passage from a female plant. It releases its proteins to find out if you are its mate! People who are allergic to that kind of pollen give a vehement negative reply. Their immune systems declare war.

People who have symptoms throughout the year are more likely to be allergic to mold spores, dust, animal danders, or chemicals such as tobacco smoke, or fumes in the home or workplace. Molds that cause allergies are small fungi. Outdoors they travel on the wind much like pollen and are more common from spring to fall. In some cases, people allergic to molds are mistakenly thought to have pollen allergies because their symptoms are not as bad in winter. Indoors, however, molds can trigger reactions at any time. Some people who are allergic to them can develop symptoms from buying foods, such as mushrooms, in a supermarket. They inhale invisible spores as they select and bag their purchase. Molds can grow on other foods, in cellars, or on stuffed animals, mattresses, furniture, and sometimes in air conditioners.

House dust is a common culprit. It can be composed of a wide array of minuscule particles, many of which can trigger allergic responses. In 1967, a group of Dutch researchers showed that some patients are allergic to mites growing in the dust. Dust mites seem to be more common in old homes, especially in countries with damp climates. It is not easy to keep a house dust-free, but most doctors advise patients with dust allergies to rid their homes of dust collectors, such as thick carpets, drapes, and upholstered furniture. There are some dust-proofing products on the market, for instance sprays that inhibit the formation of dust.

Animal dander or bird feathers create problems for many people, especially if the animals or birds are family pets living in the same home. When doctors are tracking down the cause of a patient's allergy, they may suggest that a family pet have a holiday away from the home for a few months to see if the patient's difficulty eases. It might save the family the grief of giving the pet away for good, should the patient get no better in its absence. In a British Columbia study of children attending an allergy clinic, 35 per cent were allergic to cats and 24 per cent to dogs. Studies in Finland and Arizona have shown that even among the general adolescent populations, not just young people with allergies, 15 to 20 per cent react to cat allergens and five to seven per cent to dog allergens.

One reason allergies to cats are more common than to dogs is the cat's habit of grooming itself by licking its fur. A major cat allergen, found in the saliva, is transferred to the fur and can get into the air. There is some evidence, according to the Canadian Pediatric Society, that an infant exposed to a cat during the first six months of life is more likely to develop an allergy by adolescence. However, the same has not been found true in dog allergy. And in most cases, if a child is allergic to one breed of dog, he or she will be allergic to all breeds, although the severity of allergy may vary.

Some parents think it will be all right to keep a pet if it is kept out of the allergic child's bedroom. That's better than nothing, but animal hair and dander circulate throughout a house, carried by air currents and in forced air heating systems. Sometimes there are pets in school classrooms. Parents of children with severe animal allergies would be wise to inquire and arrange for the class pet to be removed, or find ways for the child to avoid exposure to it.

Nobody develops an allergy on the first encounter with a substance. But that first exposure sensitizes an allergy-prone person to the allergen. Next time, or perhaps not until 10 encounters later, symptoms occur. It may depend on how much IgE that is able to recognize the allergen remains in the body, or on how stridently T cells order production of the antibodies.

Some people wonder if moving to a different region would eliminate their allergy. Unfortunately, that isn't always the answer. No place is free of pollen or molds. It is quite likely that the allergic person, escaping one kind of allergen, will before long become sensitive to another one in the new home town. It may be possible, however, for those with pollen allergies to leave home during the peak pollen period to avoid areas laden with the plants or trees that bother them.

Current treatment of hay fever includes antihistamine medications, which give temporary relief. Older versions of these drugs made people sleepy, and those using them were warned not to take alcoholic drinks while on them. Today, however, those unwanted side-effects can be avoided. New forms of antihistamines don't cause them. Examples of these new antihistamines are terfenadine and astemizole. They need to be taken only once or twice a day because they are long lasting.

In addition to antihistamines, or when antihistamines don't prove effective, doctors may prescribe cromolyn, sodium cromoglycate, or other decongestants to prevent nasal symptoms. Doctors tell patients not to use nose drops or sprays for too long. Extended use can cause a rebound reaction that makes the nasal passages swell and become congested, so that a patient's rhinitis is worse than before. There are also antihistamine eye-drops that give relief to those with itchy, inflamed eyes; but again, they should not be used for prolonged periods.

Topical steroids are also sometimes prescribed during the allergy season. Steroid drugs are like natural body hormones, such as cortisone. Doctors use the term "topical" when they refer to a drug that is used locally, for example, applied to the skin, or, as in the case of allergies, sprayed or inhaled into mouth or nose. Systemic steroids, on the other hand, are drugs that go through the entire body; they are injected or swallowed as pills or capsules. Steroids are powerful drugs and doctors prescribe systemic steroids with caution. Topical steroids are considered relatively safe, although some patients suffer nosebleeds or headaches. Commonly, it takes a week to a month of regular use of a topical steroid to determine its effectiveness in relieving symptoms. Examples of steroid drugs are beclomethasone, dipropionate, and flunisolide.

Natural hormones in the body may affect the degree of allergic reaction. For example, although men and women are vulnerable to the same allergens, women's symptoms often change — becoming better or worse — during menstruation, pregnancy, and menopause, when hormone levels are altered.

With skin tests, allergists try to determine the exact causes of a patient's allergies. If the allergen being tested causes an allergic response, a small red area — what we might call a hive but which doctors call a wheal and flare — appears on the skin. It may be possible to make the patient less sensitive to those substances by a series of injections of purified allergens. The shots contain tiny doses of the allergens, with the size and strength of the dose slowly increased over time. It causes the immune system to produce IgG against these substances. Doctors sometimes call this blocking IgG because these antibodies attach themselves to the allergens, blocking IgE from latching onto them. For the most part, this therapy works best against pollens and is more effective in children and young adults. The shots are only effective if the allergist has been able to pinpoint precisely the allergens that affect the patient. In many cases, that is not possible. Usually shots are given once a week at first, tapering off in frequency. Make sure you know exactly which allergens are being used if you are taking shots, and inform your doctor promptly of any adverse reactions to them. In rare instances, allergens in an injection can trigger anaphylaxis.

ASTHMA

If for any reason you've been unable to get your breath for a split second and have felt you were suffocating, you know a little about how frightening it feels to have an attack of asthma. Asthma is an ancient Greek word that means "to breathe hard." A person with asthma who has an attack feels short of breath because the inner walls of small airways, called bronchioles, become thick with fluid. They go into spasms, kinking, so they are no longer straight and fully open. At the same time, the lungs produce a thick, sticky mucus, or phlegm, plugging the airways. The person finds it difficult to breathe in fresh air, containing vital oxygen, and even more difficult to breathe out stale air, containing carbon dioxide. Wheezing, typical of asthma, occurs because air is trying to get through very narrow passages. On average, an adult breathes in about 10,000 litres of air per day and normally does so effortlessly. Yet in an asthma attack it can seem impossibly difficult.

People of either sex and of all ages have asthma. They include movie stars, like Liza Minelli and Elizabeth Taylor; politicians including a former American vice-president, Walter Mondale, and the late Theodore Roosevelt; and even a number of Olympic athletes. But it is more common in boys under the age of 14 and in men over the age of 45. Between two and three million Canadian children and about four million American children are being treated for asthma. Overall, three per cent of the population suffers from asthma.

What has your immune system got to do with asthma? Most children and about half the adults with asthma also have allergies, which, as we learned earlier in the chapter, are the result of a misguided attack by certain antibodies. Often an asthmatic person has a history from early childhood of different kinds of allergies, such as hay fever or eczema. The majority of children will grow out of their asthma by the time they are adults and may have, at most, only the occasional attack. It is possible, however, to develop asthma without having allergies. In non-allergic cases, often the cause is a respiratory virus infection or sensitivity to drugs such as Aspirin or to food additives. Non-allergic asthma tends to occur after the age of 40. A work environment that contains substances triggering asthmatic attacks can put people at risk of what is called occupational asthma.

Asthma is serious. In a severe attack, breathing can stop altogether. Each year in North America, some people die of asthma, although dramatic improvements in treatment in recent years have reduced the toll to one-third the death rate in 1960. Acute attacks can put a strain on the heart. Most of the time, however, asthmatic attacks cause no lasting damage. Although an attack is frightening to patients, who are unable to get their breath, and to the family, it can be overcome by prompt treatment, either at home if the attack is relatively mild and medication is at hand, or at the doctor's office or in hospital if symptoms are worsening despite home treatment. After the attack is over, breathing returns to normal. It is understandable that a person in the midst of an attack feels panicky. But panic can make matters much worse. One of the first things asthmatics need to learn is how to stay calm.

Doctors diagnose asthma with a variety of breathing tests to measure how easily air is exhaled and inhaled, using spirometers and flow meters, among other devices. In some cases, with the patient under careful supervision, they provoke an attack to find out which allergens cause the asthma. If the allergens are identified correctly, it may be possible to help the person avoid them. For example, if cat hair is a problem, the person would be wise not to visit friends with cats in their home but to meet them elsewhere.

At one time, it was believed that children with asthma should not be allowed to exercise. It is true that exercise can trigger an attack in an estimated 60 to 90 per cent of asthmatics. (In fact some people who don't even know it may have exercise-induced asthma. They think they are merely out of shape or that wheezing is normal after exercise.) But today allergists generally agree it is better for asthmatics to take part in sports and to learn how to keep their symptoms under control while they exercise. Being fit and active with their friends is better for them.

Researchers have demonstrated that loss of heat and water in the respiratory tract, which occurs when a person who is exercising strenuously breathes in extra volumes of air, can set off exercise-induced asthma. Asthmatics have twitchy airways — that is, they tend to go into spasms quite easily. Swimming is often considered one of the best exercises for asthmatics, because in a pool they are breathing in a warm, humid air and their airways don't lose heat and moisture.

It is also known that leukotrienes, which cause narrowing and loss of elasticity of small airways, play a part in causing the spasms; it has been suggested that loss of heat and water spurs production of leukotrienes.

Pollen in the air or cold, dry weather can increase the chance of exercise-induced asthma in susceptible people. If they are joggers, for example, they tend to get it when the weather becomes crisp. Typically, an attack begins abruptly after exercise is finished, and can last from a few minutes to two hours. In some people it doesn't show up right away, but begins four to 10 hours after exercise.

Occupational asthma has been rising rapidly in industrial societies. Literally thousands of substances used in industry may have an impact on the airways of asthma-prone people. It is a significant problem in the food industry, particularly among people constantly exposed to flour dust or to fish and seafood, or even among chefs who daily inhale particles of food, such as garlic, onion, or cinnamon. Dock workers may develop it from dust of castor beans, coffee, or cocoa. Laboratory workers are at risk, typically after two or three years, if they handle animals. There are chemicals in industrial plants manufacturing foams and adhesives, in platinum refineries from nickel salts, in plastics and resins of glue used to make plastic products, any of which can trigger occupational asthma in some people. The most common wood dust asthma is caused by red cedar. In some people red cedar asthma clears up soon after they avoid the dust. However, about half of the patients have to wait six months or more for the asthma to stop recurring, and about a third may have asthma for several years after their last exposure. Doctors who suspect some of their patients have occupational asthma may want to know where they worked previously, in order to find out if the substance causing the symptoms is present in the workplace now, or if the asthma is the result of past exposure. Even people who don't work in such industries but who live near factories or plants may inhale enough dust, over time, to get asthma; so can families of the workers, as the workers inadvertently bring it home on their shoes and clothes.

In the past 10 years, say doctors, the improvement in treatment of asthma has been so great that today 98 per cent of asthma patients are able to lead fairly normal lives. Treatment needs to be tailored to the individual patient.

To prevent asthma attacks, doctors prescribe sodium cromoglycate; it stops overly sensitive airways from reacting to allergens. Inhaled in the form of a fine powder or mist, which is administered by means of a special aerosol device or face mask, the drug is forced through the mouth or nose deep into the lungs. Ordinarily, patients use it daily to ward off attacks. When wheezing occurs, other medications are needed to open up the airways.

Possibly the most widely-used medications are broncholidators (medicine that widens the bronchioles). They are used in acute attacks for people who have occasional bouts with asthma, or for long-term treatment in people with chronic asthma.

Bronchodilators can be divided into three main classes of drugs: beta adrenergic agonists, anticholinergics, and methylxanthines. The goal of the drugs is to relax smooth muscles of the airways. Beta adrenergic agonists act on sympathetic nerves that secrete a hormone, epinephrine, which relaxes small airways. The Greek letter, beta, refers to a family of receptors located throughout the body that receive messages. Some heart drugs, known as beta blockers, should not be used by people with asthma; they act in the reverse way to beta agonists (stimulators).

Ordinarily, airway relaxation is balanced by cholinergic activity, nerve messages that constrict the airways. It may help in an asthma attack if those messages can't get through. Anticholinergics interfere with the message, countering tightening or narrowing of airways, making breathing easier.

Methylxanthines are thought to act on respiratory and diaphragm muscles, although the action is not fully understood. Among the best known bronchodilator drugs is one of the methylxanthines called theophylline, although it has many different brand names. It is a chemical related to caffeine. While it has been used for two generations, new formulas allowing slow release make effects longer lasting, and according to doctors, new, fast tests to measure blood levels have made it easier to use successfully. Beta adrenergic agonists, in the past, were worrisome because they affected more of the body than simply the lungs. Beta receptors are located in other parts of the body, including the heart; epinephrine causes the heart to speed up. Recently, drug companies have marketed new, more specific forms of these drugs, known as beta-2 agonists. They act on a select group of beta receptors, primarily in the lungs, and are usually preferred over beta-1 agonists, which also affect the heart and circulation. Examples of beta-2 agonists are salbutamol and terbutaline.

Steroids are sometimes also used in acute attacks, or for severe chronic asthma. A form of the body hormone, cortisone, steroid drugs are powerful and can have serious side-effects. They are less risky when used as inhaled drugs, which is usually the form prescribed for emergency use in an asthma crisis. A steroid is only taken as a tablet by patients who have such severe asthma that the attacks are often life-threatening.

The treatment of asthma has been improved with better inhalant devices to deliver drugs as sprays, mists, or powders. New designs in inhalers have made the drugs more effective in getting the drugs to the lungs where they are needed. In the past, inhalers tended to give out a strong jet spray that hit the back of the throat and was largely wasted; a slow puff, however, allows the medicine to reach the lungs. Inhaled drugs hold an advantage over tablets or capsules because they go directly to the lungs without affecting the whole body. A number of current medications are longer-lasting than earlier drugs, making their administration easier for patients.

As research continues to provide new understanding of allergies and asthma, new drugs to get at the trouble in different ways will become available — for example, drugs to counteract leukotriene production. Some doctors think antileukotrienes will become as familiar to us as anti-histamines. Calcium blockers may be useful, especially in preventing exercise-induced asthma or attacks set off by cold air; research is demonstrating that calcium must be present to trigger asthma attacks.

If you have asthma, you need all the information your doctor can give you about the drugs you are taking. For instance, hard exercise in summer that makes you sweat heavily could affect the blood levels of the drug theophylline. Smoking and diet can also affect the way the body handles asthma drugs.

Other factors in your life that can have an impact on your disease should be considered. For instance, a teenager who had asthma as a child but has become free of it — which often happens — will get it back again if he or she starts smoking cigarettes. Smoking will make asthma worse in almost all patients of any age. Physicians usually advise smokers who develop asthma later in life to quit; an asthma attack provides strong motivation to give up cigarettes or pipe. But if you are a smoker and quit, you may find your asthma gets worse for a while. Don't be discouraged. Doctors think that in a long-time smoker, absence of smoke chemicals in the body may temporarily confuse the immune system, which has adjusted itself to the polluted internal environment. The condition is almost certain to remedy itself fairly soon.

You will probably want to learn methods of breathing to help yourself get the necessary oxygen should you have an acute attack. Some doctors advise sitting with shoulders hunched, elbows out, and hands on knees while you take small breaths. You need information on which sports are okay for you and which are not. Usually asthmatics should avoid endurance events such as long distance running. Take a hard look at the work environment and activity required if you are considering starting a new job.

Most asthmatics learn, sometimes the hard way, not to exercise or undertake heavy physical work when they have a viral infection in the respiratory tract. You are the only one who can assume responsibility for remembering your medication and taking it at proper intervals. One asthmatic Olympic swimmer had to be pulled from a pool when he developed a severe attack because he had forgotten his medication that day. When your doctor has determined which drugs or combination of drugs you should take, ask him or her to explain the treatment as fully as possible and to tell you of anything that might change its effectiveness. If you are to take drugs through an inhaler, make sure you know how to load it, use it properly, clean it, and store it.

When people with asthma say, "I had to learn to live with it," they don't mean they merely had to accept the idea that they had a long-lasting disease and would have to make the best of it. There is a lot to learn in order to live a normal life when one has asthma. Learning all you can about your disease can put you in control of it most of the time and give you confidence that you can deal with an attack, if and when one does occur.

FOOD AND DRUG ALLERGIES

Tracking down the source of the problem in people with suspected food allergies often requires the skill of a Sherlock Holmes. It may be far from evident which foods are causing the immune system to react as if it had encountered an enemy, or even whether the reaction is an allergic one at all. The symptoms, which can range from nausea, cramps, and diarrhea in some people, to eczema or hives or asthmatic wheezing in others, can result from an array of causes. And while most people with food allergies develop the symptoms immediately, or within an hour of consuming the food that causes them trouble, others' symptoms don't appear for several hours or even days.

As in other allergies, the underlying reason for a reaction is the over-production of IgE. Substances, usually proteins, in the particular food have been erroneously identified as undesirable aliens and are attacked. Compounds, like histamine, are released causing swelling and other effects in the digestive tract or in the skin, wherever the battle is being fought, or in rare instances causing widespread, life-threatening allergic shock.

Nobody knows for sure how extensive food allergies are. One estimate puts the incidence in children at one in 12 and in adults at one or two in 100. Other experts say food allergies are not nearly as common as most people think. Babies tend to have more food allergies; some doctors think it is because food proteins are among the first foreign proteins that they encounter. Most allergists agree that milk, eggs, nuts, and shellfish are the most common culprits. Some experts add citrus fruits, tomatoes, celery, and legumes to that list. Others say that although a lot of people think they are allergic to citrus fruits, strawberries, and chocolate, these are not all that common as the causes of allergy.

Some evidence indicates that if infants can be prevented from acquiring allergies in the first six months or so, much childhood food allergy could be avoided. For that reason, a number of physicians advise breast-feeding babies for as long as possible, and waiting until they are a year old before giving them egg white; milk and egg whites are two of the most common sources of food allergens.

But breast-feeding is not a sure-fire guarantee that an infant won't be exposed to cow's milk allergens in infancy. As we learned earlier, the first exposure to an allergen doesn't cause an allergic reaction. At that time the antibodies (IgE) are merely primed. But they'll be ready to stream into action upon a later encounter. Yet doctors have seen babies who appeared to have an allergic reaction to cow's milk the first time they were given it, even after lengthy breast-feeding. Before birth, babies are able to make IgE by the 11th week of gestation and it is possible the allergens were first encountered from the mother before the baby left the womb, or that they found their way into the mother's milk after she ate milk products. However, such cases may be rare.

More recently, medical sleuths in the state of New York found that of 12 babies who reacted with hives to cow's milk after first feedings of it, most had been given infant formula containing some milk in the newborn nursery. Since then the state has required hospitals to obtain permission from both the mother and obstetrician before giving newborns supplemental feedings. This means allergy-prone families will have a better chance of keeping a child free of exposure to allergens that might well lead to allergic reactions. In some children, such sensitivity can last several years, triggering an outbreak of hives or rashes every time they consume even trace amounts of milk allergens. In certain cases, the tip-off that a baby is at risk of milk allergy is when hives appear if any milk gets on the baby's skin.

California researchers have found that many people allergic to milk are really allergic to certain proteins in it. A large percentage of these sufferers react to betalactoglobulin, which makes up about 10 per cent of milk. Others reacted to alphalactalbumin or to casein, two other milk proteins. High temperatures can alter certain proteins so that they no longer cause allergic reactions, the scientists reported, adding that some babies allergic to milk didn't have reactions if their formulas were heat processed at temperatures above 100 degrees centigrade (boiled for a period of time). It could lead to new methods of processing milk products so that some people with milk allergies don't have to avoid milk entirely. Tests are already being developed to determine which fraction of a food causes an allergy.

Many people who think they have milk allergies really

have lactose intolerance, although the symptoms, which can include cramps and diarrhea, may mimic allergy. Their difficulty with milk has nothing to do with antibodies but stems from lack of an enzyme to break down the milk sugar, lactose. A number of races lack the enzyme, including Finns, Chinese, American blacks, and North American Indians.

To pinpoint which foods are causing allergies in a patient, doctors often ask patients to keep a food diary, listing everything they eat, symptoms that subsequently arise, and the intervals between meals and symptoms. An elimination diet may be prescribed. All suspect foods are removed from the diet for a time. If symptoms disappear, the foods are added back one at a time to find out which ones make symptoms return. Those foods should then be avoided. That's easier said than done; foods such as wheat or milk are in hundreds of food products, and sometimes even a trace amount can bring on a reaction. A medical journal describes a person so allergic to peanuts that he collapsed and died minutes after eating a sandwich that had been made with a knife previously used to spread peanut butter. Babies highly sensitive to egg white have developed rashes, hives, asthmatic wheezes, or have even choked when eggs were being prepared near them. Some people have allergic reactions to food, such as celery, only if they exercise within an hour or two of eating. But they can eat it safely if they stay quiet afterwards.

People with food allergies must learn to read labels avidly. They should be wary of other foods in the same family as those to which they are sensitive. Those allergic to peanuts, for example, may also react to soy beans or other legumes. Many discover that if they are careful to avoid certain foods during the hay fever season, they can eat them at other times. Doctors advise a person who has had a reaction to a food to avoid it for six months. After that, to test themselves, they may try a small amount; however, people with severe allergies are well advised to avoid the food for the rest of their lives. Unfortunately, labels don't tell the whole story, because some foods inadvertently contain substances such as a bit of mold. A canned or frozen fruit juice, for example, might cause a reaction in a person allergic to mold while the same fruit, freshly squeezed at home, would be fine.

Food additives, rather than the food itself, may be the

trigger of an allergic reaction. Many people are allergic to tartrazine, also known as yellow dye No. 5, often used in foods and drugs. Sulfites are another common hazard. They are used as food preservatives and in drugs, and are often the cause of so-called "restaurant asthma." Several years ago, a young Toronto secretary, Elizabeth Tenser, in hospital for a routine appendectomy, was given an antibiotic containing sulfites. It nearly killed her. She couldn't breathe, going into respiratory arrest; for some time she was in intensive care. Not surprisingly, since then she has been super-cautious about any prescribed drug she takes, checking with the manufacturer to make certain it contains no sulfites. She is also keenly aware of foods that might contain her nemesis. Sulfites were often used on foods in salad bars to keep them looking fresh (that has been banned now in a number of jurisdictions — but don't take it for granted), or in potatoes to prevent them from turning brown, and they are found in some wines, beers, and soft drinks, as well as some sausage meats and dried fruits. An asthmatic Ottawa woman, who reacted severely to sulfites, died after eating zucchini bread containing dried raisins. Doctors later said sulfite used in preserving the raisins might have been at such high levels that as few as five raisins could have killed her.

We all consume small amounts of sulfite every day, but only the vulnerable few suffer any harmful consequences. Better labeling of foods and drugs in recent years has removed some of the worry for people like Tenser, providing they never let their guard down and forget to check labels or ask in restaurants. People with asthma are at the greatest risk. It is estimated that one in every 10 asthmatics is sensitive to sulfites. It is used so commonly that the average Canadian daily diet contains two to three milligrams, but a meal in a restaurant, or a helping of a sulfite-laden dish, may expose a person to a dose of sulfite many times higher. Some doctors advise patients with asthma to take along their broncho-dilators when they dine out and to take antihistamines if they develop hives or itching. Those at risk of allergic shock are also advised to carry an adrenalin kit.

Monosodium glutamate, a taste enhancer, which is responsible for what has been called "Chinese restaurant syndrome," may also set off an asthma attack, some doctors have reported. The syndrome itself is not a true allergic response but it can include headache, heart palpitations, and feelings of weakness or numbness.

Allergic reactions to drugs are common. Sometimes the response is to the active ingredient, sometimes to coloring agents or filler materials that are used in the preparations but that give no medical benefit. In the United States, some 200,000 patients in hospital suffer allergic drug reactions, according to recent estimates. Another 50,000 people taking drugs at home have allergic drug reactions severe enough to send them to hospital. Penicillin has long been known to be dangerous to people sensitive to it because it can cause anaphylactic shock. It heads the list of drugs causing allergic reactions, followed by acetylsalicylic acid (ASA or Aspirin). Many over-the-counter medicines and prescription drugs contain ASA. And in some cases, insulin or vaccines can start up an allergic response.

In certain people, reactions to drugs are delayed, showing up as blotches on the skin or hives, or fever, or swelling of various parts of the body days later. Usually the symptoms vanish within 48 hours after the drug is stopped. Dyes, used for x-ray studies, called contrast media, are also a potential hazard to some people, and so far no foolproof way has been discovered of testing patients in advance to give warning of the sensitivity. A new, safer dye has now been developed, but the old type is still used because it is less expensive. Persons who are to undergo testing that requires dye should be informed of the type of dye to be used and risk involved.

In the past few years, a number of studies have suggested links between food allergies and other ailments, such as migraine headaches, excessive sleepiness, and Crohn's disease (an inflammatory disease of the small bowel). A study in California indicated that migraines are caused, entirely or in part, by food sensitivity in about 80 per cent of cases. The researchers found that each patient in the study reacted to three or four foods; by carefully managing what they ate, almost half stayed free of headaches over nine months of follow-up. Chicago doctors say histamine may be linked to cluster headaches; these headaches come on suddenly and are excruciating, throbbing, and generally one-sided; the eye may become bloodshot and stream copiously. Sometimes they occur in clusters of three or four a day, with only short periods of relief between them. Histamine levels in the blood rise during attacks and sufferers have been found to have blood vessels that respond more strongly than normal to histamine, which makes blood vessels widen. Certain drugs, such as ergotamine and beta-blockers, act on blood vessels, preventing excessive widening (the cause of the pain); they should not be taken by people with asthma or hay fever (see the asthma section above).

Although still hotly debated, one school of thought claims that arthritis symptoms may occur as a result of food allergies, and some practitioners say eliminating certain foods from the diet eases the arthritis. However, the theory is generally discounted by most allergists. Many people believe that food allergies are a cause of behavior problems in children, but there is no hard evidence to prove it. One study, involving an assessment of overly active children whose parents claimed they were allergic to sugar, concluded there was no basis for the parents' belief. Yet another found a connection between sugar and the learning ability of some children. But sugar is a carbohydrate and carbohydrates make people sleepy, lowering mental alertness. Ear-rattling snores and falling asleep over meals may be symptoms of food allergies, some doctors believe. The kinds of food that make certain people excessively sleepy vary from person to person; a Texas study found that wheat, corn, fish, eggs, and nuts made some patients doze off. In such people, sleep-inducing foods cause increased levels of IgE, according to the study. Patients persuaded to give up those foods became less sleepy at mealtimes. Snoring may result from swelling in the soft tissue of the palate and in the nasal airways, triggered by allergens.

With both foods and drugs containing so many compounds — some added to enrich them, some to improve appearance or make them more palatable — you can see how perplexing diagnosing food allergies can be. Sometimes parents trying to discover the guilty foods in a child's diet may do more harm than good. The parents may eliminate foods from a child's diet too zealously, affecting the child's growth: every year at Toronto's Hospital for Sick Children, specialists see children who are malnourished and sick because of such restrictive diets, or who have been poisoned by overdoses of vitamins their parents have given them in an attempt to make up for the elimination of foods.

Some people drastically reduce their own diets when they heed the advice of dubious practitioners who use tests, not proven to work, and tell them they are allergic to 30 or 40 foods. Doctors say an allergy to so many foods is highly unlikely. Patients, children, and adults should follow an elimination diet designed to detect a food allergy only under the strict supervision of a qualified physician. If you suspect one particular food is your problem, there is no harm in avoiding it for a while to see if your symptoms vanish. But removing many foods for any length of time is risky. Eating a wide variety of foods is the best way to ensure that your body gets everything it needs to keep healthy.

INSECT STINGS

Written in hieroglyphics on the tomb of an Egyptian King, Menes, who died 4,600 years ago, is the information that the royal personage died of a hornet sting. It's quite probable that no year since has gone by without the sting of an insect causing some deaths. An estimated 100 North Americans die that way each year, although on average in the United States only 22 fatalities are identified on death certificates as being caused by stings, a number that has remained constant since 1950. In many cases the cause is not recognized because the person has died alone and there is no evidence of the sting, no swelling or redness at the site; allergy to the insect venom resulted in anaphylactic shock with collapse, unconsciousness, and respiratory arrest. It seems incredible that death could follow something as simple as a bee or hornet sting. Ordinarily, being stung causes no more than an "ouch." The spot gets red, swells up and hurts for a while, but is gone in a couple of hours. Sometimes the swelling may be extensive, not easing up for a day or two, or even lasting for a week. But it is when the reaction involves the whole body, causing dizziness, weakness, and nausea, that prompt treatment is essential or it may be too late.

It is startling evidence of how powerful the immune response can be. Dynamite, set off during the construction of a roadway, can clear an area for work; set off improperly, it can destroy the whole project. So with the immune system.

As in other allergic responses, IgE antibodies, formed against venom, set off the explosion. They were formed at the time of first exposure to the venom which may have occurred years before. Since 1983, doctors conducting autopsies have been able to measure venom-specific IgE antibodies in blood when investigating the death of a person from unknown causes. It has cleared up some mysterious deaths. Researchers have also investigated the incidence in the population of venom allergies. Studies of blood from blood bank donors have found that about one in 100 persons has high levels of venom-specific IgE.

Each year about one million North Americans are treated for severe sting reactions. Most of them are under the age of 20. However, a fatal reaction is more likely to occur in people over the age of 50. The insects involved include honeybees and bumblebees, yellow jackets, hornets, wasps, and some stinging ants, such as the fire ant and harvester ant. Recent articles report cases of mosquito bites causing acute attacks of asthma in people with lifelong allergies.

In the past few years, scientists have taken a major step forward in treatment. They have been able to obtain pure venom to be used for immunotherapy. Given in small doses, which are gradually increased in strength, the venom teaches vulnerable persons' immune systems to tolerate the venom, so that if stung, they will not have a wild, dangerous reaction. The unwanted reaction is averted because the person's immune system makes a different kind of antibody, IgG, to the venom and these antibodies don't cause mast cells or basophils to release their potent compounds of histamine and leukotrienes. Should a sting occur later, they are able to bind to venom allergens and rid the body of them before they encounter IgE antibodies that will detonate the dynamite cells.

Previously, products for the shots were unreliable. They were made from the whole bodies of insects. Those earlier serums are now recommended only for beekeepers who may have allergies to inhaled insect proteins. The venom for the newer kind of injections is obtained from bees by placing electric grids outside hives. When a bee alights on a grid, it gets a slight shock and stings, depositing pure venom that can be collected later. Venom from hornets and wasps is obtained directly, by dissecting venom sacs. Pure venom extracts are also used in skin tests to find out whether a person is at risk. (The old products often caused positive skin reaction tests in both normal and allergic people and were useless.) Canadian scientists at the University of Manitoba have developed a new concept of therapy. It involves coupling the venom to a chemical that seems to increase the production of protective IgG. It has been found to be effective in tests on beekeepers in Sweden who were allergic to bee venom. Its advantage over former serums is that it can be given in high doses over a short time without setting off a response by IgE antibodies.

About one-third of people who react strongly to stings have a history of allergies. Some people have a severe reaction to venom that is not an allergic reaction. They are reacting, in effect, as they would to any toxin or poison.

Doctors recommend venom immunotherapy for people who have had, in the past, a severe reaction affecting the whole body, and who have a positive response to a venom skin test. Some also advise it for people who suffer wheezing after an insect bite. They also recommend to people with allergies an emergency kit that contains measured doses of epinephrine (adrenalin) in disposable syringes.

The best thing for susceptible people to do, of course, is to avoid being stung. While 100 per cent safety can't be guaranteed, allergists offer a number of tips that can help. Don't wear perfume, hair spray, or lotions that might attract insects. The insects are also attracted by food smells, so if you are cooking outdoors, keep both the food and yourself well covered. Wear shoes or sneakers rather than sandals. Don't wear bright colors or flowery prints or black. Insects are more attracted to them than to white, green, or tan. Keep a pest spray can in your car in case a stray insect should fly in. Don't go off alone outdoors, hiking or cycling, and if you are gardening take care not to disturb wasp nests or bee hives.

Wasps build nests or mud structures under leaves and in carports or in woodpiles. Hornets' nests are grey, football-shaped structures, usually found in trees or shrubs. Yellow jackets' nests are often found in cracks of rock walls or between walls of frame buildings. Get rid of nests around your home. But don't do it yourself if you are susceptible, and don't let any susceptible person into the vicinity while the nests are being destroyed. Commercial pest sprays, used at night when the insects have returned to the nest, are effective. The person doing the spraying should wear a hat, long sleeves, work gloves, and boots or heavy shoes.

Bees leave the stinger behind after they sting, which attaches the venom sac to the skin. If you are stung by a bee, removing the stinger immediately may help. One quick scrape of the fingernail should get it out. Don't squeeze it, because that may release more venom from the sac. Some people claim vitamin B helps protect against insect stings. They may be right, say some allergists. The vitamin is excreted in sweat and the odor is unpleasant to bees and other stinging insects and so acts as a kind of repellent.

SKIN ALLERGIES

From the time we were kids, most of us were taught to watch out for poison ivy, the three-leafed weed that is one of the commonest causes of allergic skin reactions, which doctors call contact dermatitis. Poison ivy and its cousin, poison oak, are said to be the greatest cause of workers' compensation claims for skin diseases in North America. The U.S. department of agriculture's forest service, for example, reports that poison oak and ivy reactions account for 10 per cent of all time lost from the job, and on occasion, have put out of commission 30 per cent of the forest fire fighting force for two weeks. As some cottagers have learned, to their dismay, it is foolish to burn poison ivy in an attempt to get rid of it if you stand around and watch the fire. Smoke from the fire can contain particles of the plant, and if it blows into your face, you may wind up with your whole face or other unprotected parts of the body covered with the typical poison ivy rash and weeping blisters.

You can also get poison ivy second hand, so to speak. One allergist described a patient with poison ivy rash in the shape of two hands on her buttocks. Her boyfriend, it turned out, was a groundskeeper at a local golf course and had paid her a visit after clearing poison ivy from a fairway. The allergen in poison ivy or oak is urushiol, a component of sap. At the University of California, San Francisco, scientists have developed a patch test kit that can determine a person's degree of sensitivity to urushiol. The purpose is to identify extremely sensitive forest workers before they are assigned to high-risk areas.

It's pretty straightforward to discover the cause of an allergic reaction when it is something like poison ivy. But many times a great deal of sleuthing is required to identify the offender. One doctor described a patient who broke out in a nasty rash on her hands and arms every other Friday. Astute questioning uncovered the cause. The patient was employed cleaning offices, and on Thursdays, every second week, she cleaned and polished brass fittings. She was allergic to ingredients of the brass polish. Soaps, detergents, solvents, oils, lubricants, and food products can cause irritation of the skin that may be mistaken for allergic dermatitis. In some instances, which are usually difficult to diagnose, contact dermatitis can become chronic and loses the usual trademark — fiery redness and oozing — that makes doctors suspect an allergy.

The skin is often the billboard on which symptoms of allergy are displayed, with the underlying cause lying elsewhere. The itchy red rashes of eczema, particularly in babies, may be the outcome of food sensitivities. One child, whose hands broke out in a typical contact dermatitis rash every winter, was believed to be allergic to wool mitts. All sorts of mittens were tested, without success. The problem continued until the child was snowed in on a visit to her grandmother in a small northern Canadian town. Because shipments of fresh foods could not reach the town for two weeks, the youngster did not have her usual morning orange juice. Her hands cleared up. Subsequent trials of orange juice when she returned home to the city brought back the rash each time. Foods had not been suspect because the child experienced the symptoms only in winter. But in summer her family ate other local fruit, berries, and melons, for breakfast.

Hives can crop up as a result of exposure to foods, drugs, insect stings, or even sunlight, exercise, or cold exposure. Small, round hives on the surface of the skin are called urticaria. If the blotches are large and go into deeper layers of the skin, the condition is called angioedema. In certain people, hives can occur inside the body, instead of appearing on the skin. Sometimes, the exact cause is never discovered. Usually they go away within a short time, but they may recur. Sometimes, they last for more than six weeks and are considered chronic. Doctors don't take hives lightly and they try hard to track down their cause, because hives can be an advance warning that the person might suffer anaphylaxis at some time under certain conditions.

ALLERGY TESTS

In addition to interviewing patients to find when, where, and under what circumstances symptoms of allergy arise, physicians have certain tests to help them pinpoint the causes of allergies. Most familiar to people are skin tests. They're less helpful in food allergies than in allergic rhinitis, asthma, drug allergies, and insect sting allergies, although gradually tests for food are improving. The doctor pricks the skin and puts a tiny quantity of an allergen into the skin. If IgE antibodies that recognize that allergen are around, sitting on mast cells, the site will become red and raised (wheal and flare) within 15 minutes. That is called a positive skin test, indicating that patients have been exposed to the same allergen before, although they may or may not have had symptoms from the encounter. It means they have been sensitized to the allergen and may be primed for a reaction at some future meeting with it.

Usually doctors get clues from patients' histories that help them decide which allergens to use in skin tests. The doctor would be almost certain to diagnose ragweed hay fever if a person in Ontario generally had allergic rhinitis from mid-August to frost and had a positive skin test to ragweed allergen. But the skin test alone would not be conclusive proof. Another patient could also be positive for ragweed on the test but never suffer symptoms in the ragweed pollen season, and would almost surely not be allergic to ragweed.

Prick or scratch tests are quite specific, providing test allergens are available and the doctor has a reasonable idea of which substances could be implicated. For example, in testing the patient with seasonal fall symptoms, the doctor would naturally consider weed pollens as prime suspects. The tests are safe — although in an extremely rare case they can cause allergic shock — and relatively inexpensive. But they can be uncomfortable and small children may be highly distressed by them.

When an allergen is injected into the skin, it is called an intracutaneous test. These tests are more sensitive than skin prick tests and are used if the prick test can't confirm a diagnosis. Patients should not take antihistamines for at least 48 hours before the testing; some other drugs can also affect a patient's degree of sensitivity.

Another test, devised in 1968, is called RAST, which stands for radioallergosorbent test. It is a test done on a sample of blood; the only discomfort for the patient is having the blood withdrawn. The test detects specific IgE antibodies and is the only one used for patients at high risk of a severe reaction from even a minute amount of certain allergens. But it is less sensitive than skin tests. It works this way: In the test tube, a suspect allergen is added to a small amount of the patient's blood serum. If IgE antibodies specific to the allergen are present, they will bind to the allergen. That tells testers that the particular kind of IgE that they are looking for is there. To find out how much there is, other antibodies, mirror images of that particular kind of IgE, are added. These second antibodies are labeled with a radioactive material so that they can be located. They will latch onto the IgE, and the amount of IgE that has reacted with the labeled antibodies can be measured, indicating the blood levels of that particular IgE in the patient. A similar test, called ELISA, which stands for enzyme-linked immuosorbent assay, is a variation of RAST. It uses enzymes instead of radioactive material, as the measuring stick. Both tests are available in commercial kits for doctors.

While RAST has been widely used in the United States, Canadian physicians have been slower to make use of it, largely because medicare in most provinces did not quickly accept it as an insured test. It costs about 10 times as much as a skin test and the Canadian provinces were watching their pennies. Gradually, provincial health plans are putting it under their umbrellas, although with some restrictions, to stop it from being used whole hog and thus increasing health costs.

UNPROVEN TESTS AND TREATMENTS

Rapid advances in understanding and treatment of any disease can make it difficult for the public to distinguish which findings are legitimate. Unscrupulous or money-greedy practitioners are quick to prey on people. The Asthma and Allergy Foundation of America, in a bulletin to consumers sent out in 1981, warned that the potential for fraud and quackery in the diagnosis and treatment of allergic disease is great and that unproven procedures may be dangerous.

Among them is so-called urine auto-injection. Actually, the questionable therapy has been around for about 40 years but has recently made a comeback. In this procedure, an allergy patient is injected with a small amount of his or her own sterilized urine. It is hazardous because the immune system could produce antibodies against proteins in the injected urine that might attack the patient's kidneys, possibly causing severe kidney destruction.

Another test that doctors say borders on quackery is called cytotoxicity testing, leukocytoxic testing, or leukocyte antigen testing. It is also known as food sensitivity testing or Bryan's test. Like RAST, the valid test with which a lay person might confuse it, it is a test done on a sample of blood. It is supposed to determine allergies to substances, primarily food. People who are tested sometimes are told they are allergic to three dozen foods. But studies show there is no scientific basis for the test. The U.S. Food and Drug Administration says the testing should not be done because it has not been licensed. If done by anybody who is not a doctor, it is illegal.

But despite the warnings, there are reports that it is still being administered to the gullible. In 1984, storefront franchises for the testing were sold, and teams of nutritionists and nurses were sent out by test labs to tour the country testing patients at a cost of some $325 each. The test is supposed to show alterations in the shapes or numbers of white cells when the blood sample is combined with certain allergens. One of the patients tested by a team was the wife of the then president of the American Academy of Allergy and Immunology. Though she has no allergies at all, she was told she was allergic to 19 different foods.

Another dubious treatment is called provocation and neutralization. Patients are given an initial dose of an allergen, either by injection or in drops placed under the tongue. (The tongue test is also called sublingual provocative test.) They are then given a second weaker dose to neutralize or counteract any reaction. The theory that a small dose of the same substance that is causing a person trouble may overcome the problem is a basis of homeopathic medicine. Some of the practitioners who use the neutralization therapy say that a person allergic to wheat, for example, is able, after a neutralizing dose of wheat, to eat it the next day without upset. But most allergists consider such claims bogus. It is true that tolerance to an allergen can be developed with repeated allergy shots. They work because, injected into the blood, allergens tend to cause the formation of antibodies other than IgE, and in future encounters these other antibodies may mop up the allergen. But doctors don't think the tongue test accurately identifies food allergies.

Yet another is called pulse monitoring. Its proponents claim that an offensive food increases the pulse rate and that by this means patients can learn which foods to avoid. A new test involves putting a container holding an allergen near the body or on the ear lobe and measuring heart rate. Some products that are sold, including battery-operated wristwatches, are supposed to reveal allergies by measuring muscle resistance.

In general, experts say, stay away from remedies sold by mail and from practitioners promising a cure for your allergies. There is, as yet, no such thing. Vitamin therapy and health foods are commonly advertised as cures for allergies, but there is no scientific evidence that huge doses of vitamins benefit allergic people; like anybody else, they risk toxic effects of overdosing themselves with vitamins. While some health store foods may make sense if they are free of an additive to which you are allergic, or if you use such products in place of ones with ingredients you wish to avoid, you should be sure you read the labels on health foods as closely as you would read labels on all processed food products. Your immune system is guarding you from germs, but those of us with allergies must, in turn, guard our immune system as best we can from substances that lead it astray.

CHAPTER 10

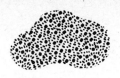

20th Century Disease

In an unusual classroom in a high school in Kitchener, Ontario, nobody wears perfume, after-shave lotion, or deodorants. There are no lead pencils and the text books have all been well-aired before being used. When it was constructed in 1985, it was probably the first classroom in North America designed for students with a condition that has come to be called 20th century disease. They suffer a variety of nasty reactions to man-made chemicals that are found almost everywhere in industrial countries, including synthetic fabrics, foods containing traces of insecticides or additives, and fumes and smells that are all around us. Kitchener is typical of most communities in having several students with the disease, some of whom were unable to attend school at all

187

and had to have tutoring at home, and others who missed so many days of school they were falling behind. As the principal of the 1,900-student school explained, these students became sick when an oil truck delivered fuel or hallways were painted or when, on a hot day, sunlight caused window drapes made of synthetic material to give off fumes.

Twentieth century disease, also called total allergy syndrome, is a baffling condition. The medical profession is of two minds about whether it really exists at all. Patients who suffer reactions to almost everything — sometimes called universal reactors — have no such doubts. Many have had to isolate themselves from society and live like hermits.

The special schoolroom is one of the first attempts to adapt a public building to the needs of such people so they may be able to live more normally. For its construction, virtually every substance normally found in a school was examined to determine whether it would offend the super-sensitive students, so that from top to bottom the remodeled classroom could be made environmentally safe. Ceramic tiles are glued in place with non-toxic cement. The walls are coated with a sealant so fumes can't escape and are covered with a non-oil-base paint. Pure cotton drapes cover the windows. The desks are old and made of wood from which any fumes have long since gone. The room is cleaned with special, non-offensive cleansers, and the water supply has a special purification system. Water-based ink is used in the students' pens; paper and books are aired for days to rid them of chemical smells. The teachers have been cautioned against using grooming products, such as hair-spray and cologne, that might trigger an episode of illness.

Nobody yet knows exactly what 20th century disease is. Indeed, there is a large segment of the medical profession that is skeptical of its even being a disease. Nothing abnormal has been found in many of the patients, despite testing with diagnostic procedures that range from cat scans to allergy tests. In one study, 50 patients were given a battery of laboratory tests to assess their immune systems, including counts of B cells and T cells and measurements of antibodies. Doctors found nothing abnormal. The patients didn't have high levels of the allergy antibodies, IgE. Skin tests, done by injecting a variety of allergens into such patients, have not indicated reactions typical of allergies. Yet doctors are seeing an increasing number of patients who seem to be allergic to the modern world.

In Canada, an organization formed by patients and their families and friends, called the Advocacy Group for the Environmentally Sensitive (AGES), says that by 1986 the number of cases had reached 15,000.

Although the condition is sometimes called total allergy syndrome, it is probably more accurately termed hypersensitivity. In the past 15 years, some physicians who call themselves clinical ecologists have focused their attention on the disease. Several hospitals in the United States and one each in Britain and Australia have devoted themselves primarily to the care of such patients. Regular hospitals, inundated as they are with chemical and synthetic disposable products, commonly are fraught with hazards for people with this inexplicable problem.

Some people with the condition have told their stories publicly in attempts to increase public understanding of the bizarre disease. One of them is a doctor — an allergy specialist. Like many of his patients, Dr. Daniel Calabrese of California, who is in his mid-30s, became hypersensitive to household fumes, molds, and synthetic products. He and his wife, who is also an allergist, turned their home outside Los Angeles into what they term an environmentally clean house. It has solar and electrical heat, instead of the natural gas formerly used, and building materials are stone, glass and wood — nothing synthetic. It has no rugs or curtains. The stove top is ceramic, because Dr. Calabrese found electric coils gave off fumes when they were heated. An oil painting on the living room wall has an air filter beside it to collect any odors the painting may give off.

Dr. Calabrese said he first noticed his strange condition in 1983 when he would lapse into periods of fatigue and moodiness and would lose all sense of time. In December of that year he spent 53 days in hospital being treated by an allergist in Chicago. It was determined he was a "universal reactor" — that he was acutely sensitive to nearly every man-made material. At that point, the Calabreses cleared their home, as far as possible, of all irritating chemicals. The doctor drinks only bottled water, which he boils again and cools before drinking. He has found one liquid cleanser to which he does not react and uses it for everything from shampooing his hair and shaving to cleaning the kitchen and doing laundry. He wears only cotton. He sleeps on a water bed, with an aluminum blanket under the cotton sheets as a barrier between himself and plastic in the water bag.

Confining himself almost totally to his home, he believes that, given time free of troublesome chemicals, his body will regain resistance and be able to cope with most things that make him ill. "Man treated the environment harshly for so many years that it is now striking back," he has said. Some clinical ecologists have suggested that people with 20th century disease are like the canaries that miners once kept below ground as an early warning of hazardous conditions. If the birds became sick or died, the miners knew the air in the mine was impure. The doctors say society should be heeding the warning being given by the most sensitive of humans among us.

A number of the patients think their disease started when they were exposed to an overload of chemicals at one point in their lives. A Canadian woman, Sandra Stonge, who is affected severely, blames it on exposure to a massive amount of insecticide in a school cafeteria where she worked and helped wash down the day after each spraying by fumigators. At the time, she was still recuperating from a bout of mononucleosis. "Severe illness combined with chemical exposure may be too much for some people," she has said. "The immune system can only handle so much." Sandra had hay fever as a teenager and later developed bronchitis and sinusitis. "However, the sensitivities I have now come from a totally different part of the immune system than do traditional allergies," she says. She thinks conventional allergies may be the first stage of the disease, followed by more generalized reactions including pain, headaches, fatigue, aches in joints and muscles, and eventually by a stage that involves being unable to think clearly and feeling depressed. The final development for some people is panic, anxiety, irrational thoughts, and mental illness.

In 1981, in hospital in Toronto, she underwent all sorts of tests, but the cause of her illness could not be identified. "I couldn't eat without getting sick, so I was entering the second stage of this whole thing. My digestive system had me in constant, excruciating pain," she told reporters later. She lost 45 pounds in six weeks. She went to a clinical ecology hospital in Chicago, spending four days in a chemical-free environment, and her symptoms cleared up. Her family altered her room at home, with changes like those made by Dr. Calabrese. Books and magazines have to be aired and her mail checked for smells before it can be given to her. A no admittance sign on the door warns away visitors because Sandra could have a reaction to something they are wearing.

Another Canadian patient, Maggie Burston, asks friends who would like to visit her to wash all their clothes, even underwear, in a health food store detergent and to wash their hair with a special shampoo that has no scent. They must not use any body lotion, face cream, deodorant, or perfume. If they agree, she might, on a good day, be able to visit with them for a couple of hours without becoming unbearably itchy or falling asleep or losing her memory. Maggie Burston, a composer of classical music, thinks the major cause of her disease was an uncontrolled common yeast infection, candida albicans. For a couple of years, there were only five or six foods she could eat without becoming terribly ill. Gradually, by carefully rotating foods, she was able to return others to her diet. But the smell of cabbage makes her faint and she falls asleep instantly if she eats lamb.

Doctors disagree over the connection between the yeast infection and 20th century disease. Yeast is normally found in the body and is harmless, but it can sometimes cause vaginal infections or white spots in the mouth commonly called thrush. Some Canadian allergists have warned that not only is it wrong to diagnose candida albicans as the cause of allergies, but that methods some practitioners use as treatment can be harmful, especially to children. One of the treatments involves giving the patient a substance containing organisms that grow in the bowel (lactobacillus acidophilus) on the grounds that candida overgrows normal flora in the digestive and respiratory tracts. One two-year-old Toronto child given the substance went into allergic shock. The boy actually had a severe milk allergy — the substance contains small amounts of milk proteins.

Malnutrition is a constant threat to universal reactors. They can tolerate so few foods that they cannot get enough to eat. They are, typically, forced to spend most of their time alone. A Toronto florist, Bob Ross, spent five years as a prisoner in his home. "You have to build an oasis. This is my cocoon. I wish I could grow wings and fly away." But he says his body was out of tune. "My immune system worked triple duty. I can notice smells much more than anyone." If he smelled a kitchen stove being turned on, his hair stood on end. Doctors could give him no explanation for it, or for why his tongue peeled, he had blurred vision, blocked ears, and was light-headed, feeling as if the room was spinning around him. During his recuperation, he had to put letters or reading material into a sealed box with a glass top or fumes from paper and ink bothered him. "This is so ridiculous why someone has to live like this," he says.

In some communities, including Toronto, parents have formed self help groups. A founder of the Toronto group, Margaret Nikiforuk, whose son is a universal reactor, says:"It's easy to think of these people as crazy. But we feel that we're just the tip of the iceberg. More and more people are succumbing to environmental stressses, environmental pollution." A public health nurse, Mrs. Nikiforuk wrote an article for other nurses in a Canadian nursing journal in which she said: "Environmental hypersensitivity is often an agonizing illness affecting the patients, the family and friends. As one patient put it, 'With this disease you lose everything; your home, your room, your schooling, your career, your friends, your hobbies.' The person who cannot tolerate an environment that to others is habitable must live like a recluse." Many of them are even cut off from outside communication; they cannot even use a telephone because of the plastics.

The mechanisms by which environmental illness arises are not yet understood. Conventional allergists argue that unless IgE antibodies are involved — and they are not — the disease cannot be considered an allergy. Clinical ecologists take the broader view that anything in the environment that a patient reacts to can be an allergy. Clinical ecologists frequently use diagnostic tests, such as the sublingual provocation test, which traditional allergists claim are unproven. (The test is described in Chapter Nine.) Controversy between the two schools of thought is likely to continue for some time. Much of the information has come from the environmentally controlled hospitals where some studies indicate that a variety of environment agents affect the immune system and the central nervous system. One doctor reports that among 400 patients treated at one such hospital in Texas, a significant number had immune system deficiencies, including a decline in T cell populations. Studies found that patients had T cells that were highly susceptible to an impact from foods, drugs, and pollutants. In particular, T suppressor cells were found to be affected. Reports in immunology journals in the past several years have described allergies that started up when people were exposed to certain substances at a time when their suppressor immune mechanisms were below normal. T suppressor cells are the ones that bring an immune response to an end once the danger from germs infecting the body is past. However, immunologists (doctors specializing in the immune system) have been unable to confirm T cell abnormalities in 20th century disease patients.

Nevertheless, from other fields of science, called immunotoxicology and immunopharmacology, a great deal is being learned about the effects of chemical agents on the immune system. One such specialist told a large meeting of allergists, "An altered immunity provokes other syndromes that may be dissociated with immune function." He listed many chemicals that suppress the immune system and alter the production of antibodies. Investigations of two situations in Japan and Taiwan found that people exposed to high levels of industrial chemicals for a substantial amount of time showed an array of changes in antibodies and helper T cells. The scientist said that sometimes the actions of drugs and chemicals in man are a health hazard and that diagnosis must include effects on the central nervous system, the endocrine system (hormones and the glands that produce them), and the immune system, because all interact.

Furthermore, many scientists are digging into another system of body defense, composed of a family of enzymes called cytochrome P450s. This system has been described as being as important in defending the body against foreign chemicals as the immune system is in defending against germs. The studies are beginning to suggest that genetic differences in people may help explain the great differences in susceptibility to adverse chemical reactions. Scientists already know that many genes govern this system, giving the body a great diversity of enzymes with which to deal with many kinds of chemicals. Toxic chemicals are not only man-made ones put into the environment in modern times but also include many natural products. The enzymes add oxygen to such compounds helping to convert them to a form that the body can more readily excrete.

For the most part, the only kind of treatments today for these patients are modeled on those used by some practitioners to treat allergies but which are generally not considered of proven value by most doctors. Patients being treated by clinical ecologists sometimes receive up to 30 shots a day to desensitize them to foods that give them symptoms; the aim is to help the body tolerate such substances. Some clinical ecologists claim to be able to rebuild immune systems with different lymphoid cell extracts, such as a solution of beef thymus. There seems little question that certain patients feel better and avoid symptoms if they are removed from environments containing gas fumes and other chemical irritants.

Twentieth century disease patients have frequently been diagnosed as having schizophrenia or other psychiatric illnesses. At one large University of Toronto teaching hospital, 18 people affected by total allergy syndrome who agreed to psychiatric consultation were all found to be suffering from recognizable psychiatric disorders. Fifteen of the 18 were well-educated women, and they ranged in age from 23 to 61. Most had been diagnosed as having 20th century disease by clinical ecologists and some had been treated at ecology hospitals in the United States. Clinical ecologists say the psychological symptoms of such patients are the result of their allergies, and would vanish if the allergies could be cleared up. Other doctors tend to believe the patients have latched onto a diagnosis more acceptable to them than one of psychiatric disorders and so cling to the idea of environmental allergies. They warn that if 20th century disease is a wrong diagnosis, people may shut themselves away from the world, wasting years of their youth, in prolonged and needless isolation.

Yet as one Canadian ecologist has said, "What these patients really represent are the medical failures. They have negative physical examinations, negative laboratory findings, and they're told to live with it. They may be operating at only 50 to 60 per cent of their potential and yet nobody can find out what's wrong with them." And an American doctor adds,

"Treatment of the total allergy syndrome is inadequate. Complete avoidance is impossible, traditional medications are insufficient and desensitization is, at best, questionable. The 20th century syndrome is fertile territory for research and may require 21st century innovations and tools for a solution."

Among people with environment-induced hypersensitivity, only five in 100 suffer the severe total syndrome. Many have mild effects. For a number of them, exposure to offending substances occurs in the workplace. And conventional allergists don't dispute the idea that modern-day sealed office buildings can breed a host of unwanted reactions. It is called the "sick-building syndrome." It stems from problems with ventilation in windowless, air-conditioned towers. Doctors have reported that in some instances, as many as 70 per cent of a building's occupants at times suffer allergic-like symptoms of eye, nose, and throat irritation, sneezing, headache, and fatigue. Because some organisms grow in humidifiers, ductwork, filters, and pumps in heating and cooling systems, outbreaks of illness in offices are sometimes referred to as "humidifier fever." The organisms cause allergic alveolitis, which is inflammation of air sacs in the lungs. Other allergic symptoms turn out to be caused by inadequate cleaning of carpets, or fumes from building materials or business machines. Rashes and itches are often caused by fiber-glass or steel wool particles that circulate through the building because of faulty ventilation. Doctors have found such fibers embedded in the soft contact lenses of workers.

Another group of people who developed arrays of symptoms similar to 20th century disease believe the problem lay inside their own mouths — in the mercury in the fillings in their teeth. One Toronto woman, Elisabeth Scott, had tingling in her hands and legs, palpitations, fatigue, abdominal pain, swollen glands, and loss of concentration and memory. "I could not remember my own phone number some days," she said later. Doctors suspected she might have the arthritic disease, lupus, and put her in hospital for investigation, but found nothing. She had psychiatric consultation, but knew she was not suffering depression. When a friend sent her an article on treatment in Sweden for such symptoms that involved ridding the patient of mercury, Mrs.

Scott went to her dentist. He agreed to replace her 20 fillings gradually. By the time a third had been changed from fillings containing mercury to non-metallic material, she'd started to improve. When all were replaced, she felt fine. Her dentist believes now the woman was hypersensitive to mercury.

Meanwhile at the University of Southern California, a dentistry professor has found the immune system can be adversely affected by mercury. His early studies show a reduction of T cells in patients with amalgam fillings that contain mercury. The American Dental Association estimates that fewer than one per cent of people are hypersensitive to mercury. Tests have been developed that can reveal if a person is allergic or hypersensitive to mercury. With the development of new filling material, such as ceramics and synthetics, the use of mercury is expected to end in future. Already some British dentists are advising that amalgam should not be used in children. If the practice of filling teeth with old-style amalgam does come to an end, it may mean our immune systems will have one less problem to deal with some day.

But for those for whom mercury is only one of dozens of substances in the world that they believe makes them feel miserable, much more knowledge is needed, if they are to be helped to lead normal lives. For certain people with the syndrome, life is not worth living at all. The organization AGES reported recently that two sufferers, desperate because doctors could not tell them what was causing their illness or offer hope of recovery, committed suicide.

CHAPTER 11

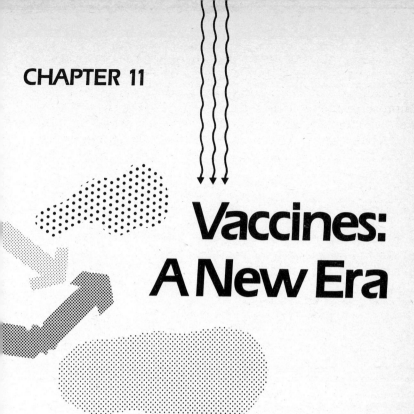

Vaccines: A New Era

A few years ago phones in children's hospitals and at the offices of family doctors began ringing incessantly with calls from worried parents. The question they all wanted answered was: "Should I have my child vaccinated against whooping cough?"

The sudden outbreak of alarm might seem strange since whooping cough vaccine has been widely used for almost 40 years in Canada and never before had there been such a mountain of concern about it. What was the big new problem?

North America, it appeared, had caught its fears from the United Kingdom. The scare had started in England a few years earlier when a British epidemiologist made public a report that said the vaccine, in some children, could cause permanent brain damage. Groups of parents made it their cause to discourage use of the vaccine. They were successful enough that whooping cough vaccination rates in Britain dropped 30 to 60 per cent. On this side of the Atlantic, an increasing number of parents also began to refuse to let their children be given the shots. Television shows featuring children who were said to be brain-damaged by the vaccine and newspaper headlines added fuel to the fire.

Canadian and American doctors grew worried. In the United States, between 1981 and 1984, the number of cases of whooping cough doubled. At the same time, lawsuits claiming damages increased to the point where one drug company, the largest producer of whooping cough vaccine in America, stopped production; the lawsuits were costing them more than they could possibly earn in profits from the product. New worries arose about a shortage.

In Britain, epidemics had followed the decline in the number of children vaccinated. It was estimated that if an epidemic comparable to Britain's happened in North America, there would be 500,000 case, and 160 deaths a year.

In England, where whooping cough immunization rates were reported to have fallen to 31 per cent of young children by 1978, there had been within four years two large epidemics of whooping cough with a total of 100,000 cases. Thirty-six of those children died. The second epidemic, in the winter of 1981-82 was worse than the first, accounting for 21 of the deaths among 85,000 cases.

Something similar happened in Japan. Two children there had died shortly after receiving the vaccine, and the age of immunization was raised to two years of age. More than 35,000 cases of whooping cough followed, with 118 deaths. The incidence of whooping cough in Japanese infants less than age two has remained at high levels, similar to levels seen prior to the vaccination's introduction.

It is true that whooping cough vaccine causes more adverse reactions than vaccines against other contagious childhood diseases. But doctors feared the alarm that parents were expressing about it might also make people reluctant to have their children given shots against the other diseases, or launch lawsuits for damages claimed to have resulted from them. In Quebec, a family sued the province for $2-million in damages on behalf of their daughter. She had suffered a brain infection causing permanent damage eight days after she was inoculated against measles at the age of five, in 1972. The case went to the Supreme Court of Canada, which found in May 1985 that the province was not liable even though it had urged parents to vaccinate their children against childhood diseases. It was the first ruling in Canada to deal with the issue. Subsequently, Quebec enacted a no-fault compensation plan for those suffering reactions to vaccines.

Below the border, however, medical malpractice and damage suits are far more frequent. Already, hundreds of claims have been filed for damages from vaccines. An Illinois family sued both the physician and the whooping cough vaccine manufacturer for damages suffered by their three-year-old daughter. The family was awarded more than $11-million in 1983 — the first major settlement involving the vaccine. Since then, Great Britain, Japan, the Netherlands, and many other European nations have set up funds to compensate vaccine-damaged victims. In North America, by 1986, only California and Quebec had such plans.

In the U.S., vaccination against childhood diseases, including whooping cough, is mandatory unless the child is excused on medical or family conscientious grounds. Some provinces in Canada — New Brunswick and Ontario were the first — require children to be vaccinated for most diseases, except for whooping cough, in order to attend school.

The nub of the problem is that no vaccine is absolutely risk-free. Yet the deaths and damages resulting from the diseases themselves are many times greater. In Canada, in 1923, exactly 20 years before whooping cough vaccine became available, 1,374 children died of the disease. Since 1970, deaths each year have totaled on average three, with no deaths some years. "The numbers of deaths and of children with permanent brain damage from whooping cough would be at least 15 times higher than those associated with the vaccine," says a top Canadian infectious disease specialist, Dr. Ron Gold, of Toronto's Hospital for Sick Children.

Later in this chapter, we'll look at each of the major contagious diseases individually. And the directory at the back of the book tells you where to write to get booklets providing immunization information.

Body Defenses

SMALLPOX

As fear over vaccines for children was spreading, a remarkable triumph for a vaccine was announced. In 1980, the World Health Organization declared the world free of smallpox. Actually, the last case had been tracked down four years earlier in a small village in Somalia, Africa, by public health sleuths from the U.S. Centers for Disease Control in Atlanta, Georgia. Since then, every suspect case has been immediately investigated. Between 1979 and 1984 the World Health Organization received reports of 179 cases of suspected smallpox. Every one turned out to be either chicken pox or a false rumor. As far as can be determined, no free smallpox virus is loose today in the world.

It is the first time that mankind has been able to rid the world of a killer disease and, although it took almost 200 years since the smallpox vaccine was developed, it stands as an amazing achievement.

The word vaccine comes from vacca (cow). In the late 1700s, a British medical student, Edward Jenner, observed that milkmaids who had had cowpox didn't come down with smallpox during epidemics, then so common in Europe. But nobody else, royalty or peasant, was protected. Queen Elizabeth I caught it in 1562 but survived. Joseph I of Austria was not so lucky. He died of it in 1731. In those centuries the death rate was appalling. In England in 1629, among every one million people, 3,000 died of smallpox. One in four who contracted the disease died. Smallpox was so contagious, spreading from person to person, that if one member of a family got it, at least half the relatives also got it. Those who lived were often horribly disfigured by pock marks, or by gangrene, which often set in.

Today it is difficult to imagine the terror that swept over communities when cases began to appear in a town. Doctors of the day knew so little about diseases, blood-letting was virtually the only treatment prescribed. Those lucky enough to catch a mild case and live didn't get it again, although no one understood why. But young children were at the mercy of the virus.

In those days, the majority of children in England had caught smallpox by the time they were seven. But in Turkey,

200

a method of protection was already in use by inserting pus or powdered scabs from a smallpox victim into the skin of other people. They usually got a mild case of the disease but their risk of death was only a fraction of the risk when infected naturally. It is said that Lady Montague, wife of the British ambassador to Constantinople (now Istanbul) in the 1780s, was the first to bring the idea to England. But only a few would consent to the treatment. It seemed too big a gamble, and furthermore, even mild cases caused by this treatment could spread to others, perhaps causing severe disease.

Early settlers to North America brought smallpox with them, as well as other contagious diseases such as typhus, cholera, and plague, all of which devastated the native populations. Indians had never encountered the smallpox virus and had no built-in protection from their immune systems. In an epidemic in 1617-19, Indians on the coast of Massachusetts were reduced to one-tenth of their former numbers. In Canada, Indian populations were so ravaged by smallpox that in 1639, the first hospital, Hôtel Dieu in Quebec, was established primarily to care for the Huron Indians.

But in 1798, Jenner announced his discovery. He could use cowpox crusts to protect people from the dread smallpox. The British Parliament hailed Jenner as a hero, rewarding him in 1802 with 10,000 pounds and making him the director of an institute for vaccination. That same year in Canada, public funds were used to buy cowpox vaccine for Indians and children, possibly planting the seeds for a Canadian philosophy on health care that was to blossom more than 150 years later into a national, universal medicare program, whereby public funds pay for care for all Canadian citizens.

Jenner's vaccine was given directly from one person to another, from arm to arm. The major change since then has been the way the vaccine is produced and injected. Otherwise, it is much the same as it was then, a material made with the virus that causes cowpox. Now we know, however, that the cowpox virus and the smallpox virus are so similar in the eyes of the human immune system that our memory cells, taught by the vaccine to recognize cowpox, were prepared to muster troops of immune cells instantly should a smallpox virus arrive.

By the middle of this century, the dream of ridding the world of smallpox had inspired public health doctors. In 1966 the World Health Organization set elimination of smallpox as its global goal. But those who believed the goal could be reached appeared unduly optimistic. At the time, 10 to 15 million cases in the world were still being reported per year — and many countries were not reporting more than a tiny fraction of the cases actually occurring. How could the dream ever come true in our lifetime? Yet by 1972, only six countries still harbored the killer virus and four years later it was gone.

Today in North America the general public is no longer vaccinated against smallpox. Proof of smallpox vaccination isn't needed for international travel. In 1983, the last licensed producer of the vaccine in the U.S. discontinued distribution of the vaccine to civilians. Members of the Canadian Armed Forces and U.S. military personnel, however, are still routinely vaccinated, and the Centers for Disease Control provides the vaccine for laboratory workers at risk because of research involving the smallpox virus or other similar viruses. Nevertheless, public health doctors dare not let down their guard. Should the virus ever surface again, it must be stopped in its tracks at once. If not, huge populations never vaccinated will be as vulnerable as newborn babes.

But today the chance of encountering the disease is so small that getting a vaccination is riskier. Once in a while, cowpox, also called vaccinia, can develop. It is also possible — there have been a few cases — in which a newly vaccinated military person passed cowpox on to a close contact. One such case occurred in Newfoundland in 1981 and another in Louisiana in 1983. The cases indicate a potential for trouble should there be accidental spread among people for whom any infectious disease is dangerous. Cowpox, of course, is not deadly like smallpox and can be treated with an immune globulin. People who have never been vaccinated, however, would be wise to protect themselves by avoiding close or intimate contact with any person who has been recently vaccinated. In particular, a newly vaccinated person should stay away from children under one year of age, from people with eczema, and from those who have conditions that make their immune systems deficient, including inherited conditions. They should avoid people being treated for cancer or patients who are receiving anti-rejection therapy following transplants or anyone with diseases, such as AIDS, that destroy body defenses.

Eventually even the symbolic reminder of smallpox most of us wear today may disappear: future generations may never have reason to bear the scar of smallpox vaccination on thigh or arm so familiar to all but the youngest among us now.

Today researchers are investigating the cowpox virus vaccine as a vehicle to use in the making of a vaccine that would work against a broad spectrum of diseases. The idea is to insert into its genes (its blueprint) other genes that will produce molecules (antigens) of other viruses. When the vaccine is injected into the body, the immune system will make antibodies not only against the cowpox virus but also against the other viruses. By early 1985, researchers at the New York Department of Health and at the U.S. National Institutes of Health had tested such hybrid vaccines in animals. One was a cowpox vaccine modified to protect against influenza, hepatitis, and herpes, while the other, tested in chimps, was a cowpox virus containing just hepatitis genes. While there are many problems and doubts about the approach, the World Health Organization has approved continued research. Many new vaccines are in the pipeline.

This is only one example of what is promising to be a whole new vaccine era. But before we get to that part of the vaccine story, let's look at the vaccines we already have on hand.

The first shot that babies get, starting at two months, is a vaccine that protects them against diphtheria, whooping cough, tetanus, and poliomyelitis. The medical name for whooping cough is pertussis and the vaccine is commonly referred to as DPT-Polio. Babies are given additional shots of this vaccine at four months and six months. In their second year they get one more, usually at 18 months, and one additional booster at four to six years of age.

POLIO

Maybe you remember or have heard your parents talking about the days when polio so frightened people that children were not allowed to go to swimming pools or to crowded places such as big fairs like the Canadian National Exhibition. In the 1930s and 40s, few cities or neighborhoods escaped the sorrow of deaths among children who caught the virus, or more correctly one of the viruses — there are three versions. Summer and fall were the most common times for them to spread. Epidemics occurred because most people who caught the virus didn't know it and unwittingly spread it to others. In about one per cent of those infected, however, the virus was able to get into the brain or nervous system leaving victims disabled, paralysed, and sometimes unable to breathe on their own. Hospitals became home to many people who needed a machine, then called an iron lung, to help them breathe. Many others, including late U.S. president Franklin D. Roosevelt went through life with crippled legs.

Polio epidemics first began to appear toward the end of the last century, first in Scandanavia, then the U.S., and later in other parts of the world. In countries with primitive sanitation, polio primarily strikes children before the age of four. In developed countries, with better hygiene, exposure to the viruses is delayed; at the same time, however, a larger proportion of the population remains susceptible, increasing the chance of an epidemic.

For about 75 years, polio viruses had things pretty much their own way. We didn't know how to stop them from spreading. Yet within a shorter time than anyone could have dreamed, poliomyelitis was to be tamed into submission. In 1955, Dr. Jonas Salk of the U.S. presented the world with a vaccine. It was made with virus treated with a chemical, formulin, that prevented it from causing the disease. While the number of cases in North America began to drop, the vaccine didn't stop all polio. Epidemics still occurred, even among many people who had been vaccinated. The vaccine was not foolproof. The last major epidemic in Canada, with 1,887 cases, struck in 1959. Three years after that, a new kind of vaccine became available. Developed by another American physician, Dr. Albert Sabin, it was made with live but weakened virus. In 1964, in the U.S., only 91 cases were reported. In the 1970s in Canada, there were only three cases a year.

While polio has faded as a threat to children in industrialized nations, that is far from true in the Third World. One of the people who have taken on a mission to try to eliminate polio world-wide is James Roosevelt, eldest son of the late U.S. president. On speaking tours, he reminds his audience that 40,000 Third World children still die of polio every day. In three days, he points out, the number equals the death toll of the nuclear bomb dropped on Hiroshima in World War II. Since 1974, the World Health Organization has undertaken an intense program of vaccination globally and in mid-1985 reported that 40 million infants, who in 1984 survived to age one in Third World nations, had been vaccinated. That was eight times better than when the program began, but there is still a long way to go. Fewer than half of 100 million children who needed vaccination that year got it.

Vaccines may not have brought polio to its knees throughout the world yet. But for three days in 1985, one day in each of three months, they did bring about a minor miracle. On those days the war stopped in San Salvador to allow another kind of army, made up of health workers and trained volunteers, to go safely about the country immunizing children with DPT-polio and measles vaccines.

Meantime in Canada and other western nations, a new problem resulting from polio began to emerge. Many people here who had polio 30 years ago or more, were reporting a recurrence of symptoms similar to the ones they had suffered earlier, such as muscle pain, fatigue, pain in the joints, respiratory problems, and restricted use of arms and legs. In Ontario, Canada, the health ministry estimated that in 1985 some 5,500 people were affected by this perplexing post-polio condition. The average age of onset was 43 years.

Research at the U.S. National Institutes of Health has disclosed that the new disease may affect a specific muscle but not necessarily one that had originally been affected by polio. Scientists conducting a survey of some groups among the 300,000 people still alive today who had polio years ago, estimate that the late recurrence of symptoms strikes about 15 per cent of them. Doctors say that those affected need not fear

that they have a full-blown case of polio again. The polio
echo is not life-threatening nor will it progress to the point
where it is incapacitating. They also say it is not, as some
people have suggested, linked to another paralysing disease
called amyotrophic lateral sclerosis, called more commonly
Lou Gehrig's disease. In the directory at the back of the book
you will find an address where you can obtain a handbook on
the late effects of polio, written for survivors and physicians.

In general, this is what you need to know about polio
vaccines:

- Either of the two vaccines, the Salk inactivated poliomyelitis vaccine or the Sabin live oral polio virus vaccine,
  or both, may be used. It depends on the public health
  policy in your region. Both are effective.

- If you are the parent of a baby who is to be vaccinated with
  the live vaccine (Sabin) and you have not been vaccinated
  yourself, you would be wise to get a series of shots of the
  Salk inactivated vaccine. Your baby may shed viruses in
  bowel movements as a consequence of the action of the
  vaccine and when you diaper and bathe your child you
  might become infected. Of six cases of polio in the U.S. in
  1982 and 1983, five were of unvaccinated parents whose
  infants had recently been given the live oral vaccine.
  Inactivated Salk vaccine is recommended for adults because
  the risk of a vaccine-related viral infection is higher in
  adults than in children, though even in adults the risk is
  small.

- Get a vaccination if you are going to be traveling to a part
  of the world where polio is still widespread. Ordinarily,
  vaccination requires three doses of inactivated Salk at
  intervals of one to two months, with a follow-up dose
  several months to a year later. If you haven't time for a full
  course, two doses, four weeks apart, are advised or a single
  dose of live vaccine if the time before departure is less than
  four weeks.

- If you began, but did not complete, a course of
  immunization, you should only get the remaining doses,
  preferably of the same kind of vaccine. There is no need to
  start at the beginning, no matter how long the interval has
  been.

- In rare instances, the live oral vaccine has caused temporary
  paralysis. During the past 20 years in Canada such

instances have occurred once per 4.8 million doses given. In the U.S., where 20,000 cases of polio a year were reported before vaccines were available, there have been less than 15 cases per year for the last decade and all appear to be vaccine-related. The U.S. Immunization Practices Advisory Committee recommends live oral vaccine for children. A new killed vaccine is being tested, however. It looks more effective than the Salk version and requires fewer injections. If it lives up to its promise, it will become the preferred vaccine for all.

DIPHTHERIA

Sixty years ago in Canada, diphtheria was widely feared. Some 9,000 cases occurred each year and about 10 per cent of the patients died, most of them the youngest and oldest people. It is caused by bacteria that produce a toxin. The vaccine is made with the toxin that has had its fangs pulled but which brings about the same immune system response as the disease-causing toxin. Since routine vaccination of infants and children began more than 40 years ago, the number of cases has dropped dramatically. Eleven were reported in 1982 in Canada. In the U.S., in 1921, there were 200,000 cases, but by the 1980s it had become rare and the few cases still seen were among adults never immunized. But it hasn't been entirely wiped out of the country. There are still carriers who have no symptoms themselves. Because of that, the continued program of immunization is important.

Usually the protective material, diphtheria toxoid, is given to babies, combined with protection against whooping cough and tetanus, with three initial doses, a fourth dose a year later, and a booster prior to starting school. Thereafter, boosters are given every 10 years. For children over the age of seven and adults, the vaccine given does not contain whooping cough vaccine and has somewhat less diphtheria toxoid. It's given in two doses eight weeks apart with a third dose a year later.

Recently, a potentially exciting use for diphtheria toxin has been discovered. Scientists can manipulate the genes of diphtheria bacteria so that the toxin produced will only affect pigment cells. One molecule of the toxin is enough to kill a cell. Tests are under way to find out if this new form of toxin is effective treatment for malignant melanoma, cancer of the pigment cells, the most serious kind of skin cancer.

Here's what you need to know to protect yourself and your family from diphtheria:

- Adults should get a booster shot of the adult-style preparation every 10 years.
- Diphtheria toxoid may cause a local reaction at the site of injection and fever in older children or adults, but seldom results in really serious adverse reactions.
- A person who has had diphtheria does not necessarily escape the disease again. If a person does get diphtheria, a complete course of diphtheria toxoid should be given during convalescence. If there is a case of diphtheria to which you or another family member may have been exposed in a classroom or household, a dose of toxoid, appropriate for the age of the exposed person, is advised.

TETANUS

Like diphtheria, tetanus has declined remarkably in the past 40 years. About 20 people a year in Canada require hospital care as a result of tetanus, and in the years between 1980 and 1985 seven people died, five of them elderly. The decline in the number of cases began even before the start of immunization with tetanus toxoid, thanks to better hygiene and better maternity care. But in the Third World, a million newborns still die of tetanus every year.

Also like diphtheria, tetanus is caused by a toxin produced by an organism. There is no way of getting rid of the organism because it is found everywhere including in soil and animal feces, and it produces spores that can live for years. Often called lockjaw, tetanus can follow even trivial wounds. People who receive a wound, even if it seems minor and is clean, would be well advised to have a booster shot if they are uncertain about previous tetanus immunization or if the last shot was more than five years ago. Doctors advise that everybody, except those who suffered a serious side-effect from a previous dose, should get a routine booster shot every 10 years — but not more frequently or there may be adverse reactions.

WHOOPING COUGH (Pertussis)

The upsetting fears about whooping cough vaccine described earlier have had one happy outcome. They have spurred new research designed to develop better and more effective vaccines. Some of them are already being tested in groups of Canadian and American children. One new vaccine, developed in Japan, has been in use in children at two years of age for more than four years; there were adverse nervous system reactions in only four cases, among eight million vaccinations. It will be a few years, however, before the safety and effectiveness of the new kind of vaccine in infants is determined.

Whooping cough is caused by bacteria that spread in droplets ejected by coughing. Its chief victims are babies. The death rate among young infants is as high as one in 250 cases. That's why the vaccine is given so early in life, starting even at two months in premature infants. It can seem like a cold when it begins. It gets its name from the "whoop" sound patients make as they try to breathe in after a series of coughs. Symptoms seem worse at night, when babies may look blue and vomit. The cough may return during convalescence and can go on for weeks or even months after the worst, acute stage is over. Brain damage can occur when the child cannot get its breath and oxygen fails to reach the brain. It can cause convulsions or pneumonia.

Before 1981, the vaccine DPT, which contains killed pertussis organisms, was in a fluid that was injected under the skin. But now, in Canada, it is given in a form called adsorbed — this is, it is injected into a muscle. Some doctors say parents complain more frequently about redness and swelling at the injection site and report more crying and irritability in their children after injections with the adsorbed vaccine, but a large study of some 1,600 families conducted by the British Columbia health ministry found the reverse. The adsorbed vaccine is more effective in triggering antibody production in the children. It is usually injected into the thigh. About 10 per cent of children seem to have no reaction at all. But the vast majority of reactions are relatively mild and don't last more than a few days.

Parents should contact the child's doctor, however, if

there is high-pitched, persistent crying that goes on for more than three hours, if the child seems excessively sleepy and difficult to arouse, if the child is limp and pale, or if the child's temperature is higher than 103 degrees. One in about 300 children develops a high fever and cries for prolonged periods. In rare instances, once in about 100,000 injections, a child will develop brain inflammation. Once in 300,000 cases, permanent brain damage occurs. Yet the risks of the disease are much greater. The risk of brain inflammation from the disease itself is between one in 1,000 and one in 4,000. The risk of permanent brain damage is one in 2,000 to one in 8,000. Pediatric associations in both Canada and the U.S. have issued statements informing families of the importance of having babies protected against whooping cough. After the age of seven, the disease is not such a hazard. Adults may get whooping cough and think it is only a cold with a nasty cough, which hangs on and on.

Children who have had whooping cough shots during infancy require a booster shot before starting school. In Canada, even in provinces in which vaccinations against childhood diseases are required before a child starts school, whooping cough vaccination is not compulsory. However, it may be required for children who are to attend licensed day-care centers.

MEASLES, MUMPS, AND RUBELLA

Measles

The day may be coming when there will not be a single case of measles in North America. We're heading in that direction. Vaccines have been in widespread use for more than 20 years. In many jurisdictions they are now mandatory for school children unless they are exempted on medical or religious grounds. Time was when we could expect to see large outbreaks of measles about every three years. The disease used to be far more serious than most of us who caught measles as children ever realized. About one in every 1,000 patients developed brain inflammation and many were left mentally retarded. Thousands of children got pneumonia or were left hard of hearing for life. And one person in every 3,000 who got measles died.

Today, children are vaccinated after their first birthday, usually with a vaccine that also protects them against mumps and rubella. Sometimes, when a baby is at high risk of catching measles during the first year of life, vaccination is recommended even earlier. Before the age of one, however, vaccination will not provide a long-lasting or lifetime protection — the child's immune system is not mature enough. Over the years since the mid-1960s, several different types of vaccine have been used. But in Canada, the kind routinely used today is made with a live, weakened virus. It has been shown to produce antibodies against measles that last for at least 15 years. In general, one shot is all you need of the live virus material. However, people of any age who were vaccinated with the killed virus variety may require re-vaccination.

In 1934 there were 83,000 cases of measles in Canada. Compare that with the 1980s, where on average, 1,000 to 2,000 cases are reported, and you can see the enormous strides that have been made. But we can't be complacent. Unexpectedly, in 1986, Canada had an epidemic; by August, 14,000 cases had been reported, with British Columbia the hardest hit with 7,000 cases. Nearly half of the patients were between the ages of 15 years and 19 years. Public health authorities said many Canadians in this age group may have missed vaccination as young children. Widespread use of measles vaccines began in the early 1970s. In the U.S., in the past couple of years, clusters of cases cropped up among older students, especially those on college campuses. In mid-1985, the Centers for Disease Control reported that 25 campuses in 14 states had experienced outbreaks, more than six times the number of clusters that had occurred in the first six months of the previous year. Some students had been traveling abroad and apparently brought home the virus, spreading it to classmates. The problem is the same as in Canada: it seems that these university-age students, many of them born in the 1960s when vaccines were new and not compulsory, were never vaccinated and did not catch measles as kids. Some may have been vaccinated with killed vaccines and never re-vaccinated. For all these reasons, it is estimated that some 5 to 15 per cent of college students are still susceptible and that their risk increases when they congregate in large numbers on campuses. It has been recommended that university students be required to provide proof of immunization.

If you were born before 1957 you probably don't need vaccination against measles. You almost certainly encountered the wild bug. But younger people who never had a confirmed case of measles, and have not been vaccinated with live virus vaccine, would be well advised to undergo a test to see if they have measles antibodies. If not, a vaccination makes good sense. For those who are vulnerable and are exposed to measles, immunization within 72 hours of the exposure is usually preventative.

There can be adverse reactions such as fever or rash. Some people have a reaction to eggs, and these persons may develop hives or swelling of the mouth after vaccination. The virus used to make the vaccine is grown in duck embryos. In rare cases, the reaction to egg protein in the vaccine can be severe, creating difficulty in breathing and a drop in blood pressure. Children who have severe allergic reactions after eating eggs should be carefully tested by an allergy specialist prior to receiving the measles vaccine.

Brain inflammation (encephalitis) occurs once in a million doses, which is a thousand times less often with the vaccine than with the disease. And a fatal complication called subacute sclerosing panencephalitis, once seen as an aftermath of measles, has almost disappeared in North America since the introduction of vaccines.

Several hundred cases of a different measles syndrome have been reported in young adults who have been vaccinated with the killed or inactivated measles vaccine used prior to 1970. These people have developed this unusual condition after coming in contact with someone with ordinary measles. Sometimes doctors don't recognize the root of the illness. It can baffle them because it looks like pneumonia. However, doctors say that the patients recover without treatment and there is no evidence they are contagious or will get it again.

As with other contagious childhood diseases, measles is still rampant in underdeveloped countries, killing 1.5 million children in 1984. Every minute, somewhere in the world, measles kills three children and disables three more. Babies six to nine months of age are at extremely high risk, and cannot be protected because it is too early for them to be vaccinated effectively with regular vaccines. The solution may lie in a new spray vaccine, administered into the nose with a nebulizer or by a mask. Early tests suggest vaccine breathed in may protect babies at an earlier age.

Mumps

The number of cases of mumps in the United States has dropped by 90 per cent since 1968 when the mumps vaccine became available. In Canada, we don't know the national rate because mumps is not a reportable disease in some parts of the country, but it is likely the picture is similar. Many people are infected with the mumps virus and never know it, while about one in 10 infected persons develops meningitis or has complications that can include temporary deafness as a result of damage to a nerve involved in hearing. If mumps is caught by adults, 15 to 25 per cent of men and 5 per cent of women may suffer infection in reproductive organs, which can impair fertility. But sterility is uncommon, Usually only one side of the body is involved, which means that the other ovary or testis (testicle) continues to function normally, and the person is not infertile.

Usually vaccination against mumps is given in combination with measles and rubella protection and a single shot is all you need. The three-way vaccine is given around the age of one. Children, especially boys, who didn't get it as babies and have not had mumps, should be given mumps vaccine at puberty or, if it is too late for that, as young adults. Children who have allergies to eggs and experience symptoms such as hives, swelling of the throat, or difficulty in breathing, should not get mumps vaccine. As mentioned, it is produced with viruses grown in cells from duck embryo tissue. Doctors also caution that people who have had previous reactions to the drug neomycin should not be given mumps vaccine, which contains small amounts of the drug. However, those with allergies to chickens or feathers need not fear a bad reaction from the vaccine on that account and may be vaccinated.

Rubella

In the summer of 1984, a group in Toronto that opposed abortion set up a hue and cry over rubella vaccine. It was, said members of the group, made of tissue from aborted fetuses. They said that vaccine manufacturers were making a profit from abortions and therefore probably encouraging them. The gruesome picture they painted upset people. Ironically, the group came close to shooting itself in the foot. If its campaign against the vaccine had succeeded, it might well have increased the demand for abortions.

Rubella does its worst damage to unborn babies in the first three months of pregnancy and in many cases abortions were sought by women who got rubella in those critical months. "The use of rubella vaccine has prevented thousands of cases of the congenital rubella syndrome and has prevented countless abortions that would have been performed because of rubella infections in early pregnancy," said a statement issued on behalf of the Canadian Pediatric Society by Dr. Victor Marchessault of Ottawa. The syndrome involves deafness, blindness, mental retardation, and physical handicaps.

The fuss about the vaccine stemmed from the fact that rubella viruses are grown within human cells, in order to get large amounts of the virus needed to make vaccines. The cells are grown in the laboratory in bottles of nutrient fluids, and a weakened virus is added and allowed to produce many more viruses. The viruses are then separated from the cells and purified to make the vaccine. While ordinary human cells don't grow well in the laboratory, fetal cells do. The cells used as rubella virus incubators are fetal cells that were taken from the lung of an aborted fetus in Sweden in 1964. That lung tissue provided a line of cells that has been kept growing continuously ever since and which is used to produce not only rubella virus, but rabies and polio viruses for vaccine production. The protest group was mistaken in thinking cells are obtained for vaccines from newly aborted fetuses. It was also mistaken in giving the impression that abortions are being done for industrial purposes.

Fifty years ago some 70,000 cases of rubella in one year

were reported in Canada. Vaccination programs began in the early 1970s and since then the number of cases has declined substantially. Epidemics that once occurred every three to 10 years have been curbed. The U.S. federal department of health and welfare has reported an overall decrease of 98.7 per cent in 1984 compared with pre-vaccination days. Nevertheless, babies with the rubella syndrome are still being born because some 10 to 20 of every 100 women in child-bearing years are still susceptible to the virus. That isn't so much different from the percentage of women who had never had rubella and therefore were at risk before the vaccine was devised.

In Canada, different strategies were tried initially by different provinces. Seven provinces decided to vaccinate all one-year-old children. Three chose to focus on girls just before they reached puberty. After a decade, little difference in the benefits between programs aimed at one age group or the other could be seen, but a national policy was recommended to speed up prevention of the devastating problem in babies infected in the womb. In 1983, across Canada, all provinces began vaccinating one-year-olds, and six provinces routinely gave shots to girl prior to puberty, regardless of whether or not they had been immunized as babies.

Every woman would be wise, before she starts having a family, to be sure she has rubella antibodies protecting her from the disease. Doctors recommend that all women have one test for rubella antibodies prior to or during their first pregnancy. If a woman is already pregnant, and has no protection, she should *not* be vaccinated until after the baby is born. But she will want to take extra care not to come in contact with anybody with the disease.

In Britain, in 1983, Diana, Princess of Wales, helped launch a campaign urging all girls between 10 and 14 years to get vaccinated and all adult women to be tested and vaccinated if necessary. A National Rubella Council was established, with Diana, wife of Prince Charles, as its patron. A record card, resembling a credit card, was given to every girl vaccinated. Within a year, reports coming in from some regions indicated a huge jump in the percentage of young girls vaccinated, topping 93 per cent in most places.

Rubella is a mild disease in children, and it wouldn't be urgent to keep them from getting it if it were not for the risk to unborn babies. But pregnant women often have school-age children who, if they haven't been vaccinated, bring the virus home. Protecting youngsters is really an indirect way of protecting mothers.

All adolescent girls and fertile women are strongly urged to be vaccinated unless they have documented proof of having already been vaccinated. Nothing indicates that a repeat vaccination will do any harm should they already have rubella antibodies in their bodies and not know it. Women should put off pregnancy for at least three months after vaccination. Although vaccination should not be given a pregnant woman, it is safe to vaccinate mothers who are breastfeeding immediately following pregnancy. Viruses may appear in breast milk, but there are no known cases in which it caused illness in the babies.

It has been realized in recent years that children born with the rubella syndrome can continue to harbor the virus in brain, thyroid gland, other organs, or in the white cells of their immune system. As they get older and become young adults, many of them will develop a whole new range of disorders. Doctors have found that four in ten of them will have problems with insulin production and may develop diabetes and that others will develop diseases in which the immune system turns against the body.

CHICKEN POX

In most normal children, although chicken pox looks miserable, it is not fraught with serious complications. It is caused by the varicella virus. The virus was identified more than 30 years ago. Later it was found that the chicken pox virus and the zoster virus, which causes shingles, are identical. Doctors have suggested that cases of shingles in adults are caused by chicken pox viruses that had remained, silent and hidden, in their bodies for years. In newborns, chicken pox can be a frightening infection. It can be life-threatening if babies catch it from their mothers within five days before they are born or the first couple of days afterward. During that time, the infant is devoid of protection. The infected baby is usually treated with a human immune globulin made from blood plasma of people who have natural high antibody levels and with specific antiviral drugs such as acyclovir. Earlier in pregnancy, the mother's antibodies provide a defense and the baby will be fine. Once a person has had chicken pox, there is slight chance of getting it again. But it can happen, if the first case was mild and occurred in infancy. Outside of highly sophisticated laboratories, tests to determine if a person has antibodies against chicken pox are not terribly accurate.

While vaccines against other childhood diseases were developed shortly after discovering the virus or toxin that caused the disease, for 20 years there was little research aimed at producing a chicken pox vaccine. It wasn't a serious enough ailment in most children. But it was soon recognized, as drug treatments were developed for cancers and to prevent rejection of transplanted organs, that for such patients chicken pox was no trivial matter. The drugs damped down the immune system, hobbling its ability to squelch the virus. A number of chicken pox vaccines were made experimentally, and in 1974, the first vaccine made with a weakened live virus was created. Called the Oka strain, it has been the most widely tested and found to be safe and effective. Most important, it is safe to use in children and adults with leukemia whose immune systems are suppressed by drug therapy, and in other persons whose defenses for various reasons, aren't up to snuff.

Until 1984, however, it had been tried only in people who were at high risk of getting chicken pox because they had been exposed to the virus. Since then, it has been tested and found highly effective in protecting against the natural disease in healthy children who had not yet been exposed to chicken pox. The first big trial took place at the University of Pennsylvania. The vaccine was developed in Japan and is expected to be available for routine immunization of healthy children fairly soon. Doctors say it would probably be given during a child's second year, at 15 or 18 months, along with measles-mumps-rubella immunization. It is still not known, however, how long the children who were vaccinated will remain protected; only time will tell.

Chicken pox may not be a major hazard to a healthy youngster, but it has economic implications, especially for many families with a single parent or in which both parents work. In the U.S., it is estimated to cost $400-million a year, largely in lost wages of parents who must stay off work to look after the children. Until the vaccine becomes widely available, there is no way to prevent chicken pox from spreading from child to child in schools or day-care centers.

Meantime, the best protection for susceptible children, who are sick with other diseases and who have never had chicken pox, is to give them a preparation containing antibodies. These are made from antibodies obtained from the blood of people who had chicken pox and mounted a strong defense. The preparation is called varicella-zoster immune globulin. Giving a person antibodies from others, instead of stimulating them to produce their own, is called passive immunization. Healthy children don't need it, but it should be given, within 96 hours, to immune-suppressed children if they have been playing indoors for an hour or so with a contagious child. If your child is in hospital, he or she will probably be given the globulin if another child in the same room is found to have chicken pox. Premature babies, whose mothers may not have had chicken pox, should also get the globulin. In Canada, it is available through the Canadian Red Cross.

HEPATITIS

In February 1985, a prominent Toronto surgeon operating on a patient in a major downtown hospital jabbed his gloved finger with a needle. Apparently thinking little about it, he took no steps to ward off infection that might result. Two months later, the surgeon was dead of hepatitis B.

Shock waves rolled through the community, particularly jolting his colleagues in all hospitals in the province. The tragedy, as they knew, need not have happened. For three years, a vaccine against this form of hepatitis had been available and hospital workers whose jobs involved coming into contact with blood of patients had been urged to get the shots. Few of them had bothered. A year earlier, a nurse in Michigan had also died of hepatitis without even pricking her finger. The virus had probably gained entry to her blood stream through a tiny, unnoticed cut.

The kind of hepatitis they developed, called hepatitis B, was once known as serum hepatitis. There are three other kinds, each caused by different organisms. It is estimated that every year in North America more than 200,000 persons become infected with hepatitis B. One-third of them will either have no signs of disease or what they think is a mild flu-like illness. But one-quarter of them will become yellowed with jaundice, indicating that the liver is seriously affected, and more than 10,000 of this group will wind up in hospital. Furthermore, six to 10 of every 100 of those infected will become carriers, able to spread the disease to their lovers or, from their blood, to health care workers. More than 200 million people world-wide are carriers: they have chronic hepatitis B infections, never entirely ridding their bodies of viral particles.

For most of us in North America, the risk of getting hepatitis B is pretty small. But there are groups of people, eleven such groups in all, who are at high risk. Like AIDS, hepatitis B is spread by sexual contact, by sharing needles to inject drugs, and through blood or blood products. Blood donated for transfusions or used to provide blood products is screened so there is virtually no danger today of catching hepatitis B that way.

However, street-drug users who inject the drugs are at high risk. Studies have shown that one-third will have been infected within two years of beginning drug use. They account for 15 per cent of all cases of hepatitis B.

Homosexual males comprise 21 per cent of all cases, and their chance of getting hepatitis B within the first year that they become sexually active is 20 per cent. Sexual contacts of heterosexual carriers form another 15 per cent of cases, while health workers add another 6 per cent. Babies born to women who are carriers will be infected nine times out of ten and 90 per cent of those babies will be carriers. Tragically, that increases dramatically — to one in four — their chances of dying of liver cancer. Chronically infected people frequently develop liver cancer or cirrhosis of the liver, another potentially fatal disease. In fact, 80 per cent of liver cancer is blamed on chronic hepatitis B infections, and some medical specialists have said that hepatitis B vaccine could be considered the first vaccine to prevent a form of cancer.

That gives you an idea of how important vaccination against hepatitis B is for these particular groups of people. Others at greater than average risk include immigrants from

Southeast Asia, parts of Africa and the Pacific Islands, and mentally retarded young people who live in institutions.

Three kinds of vaccine are available on the world market: one developed at the Institut Pasteur in France, a Dutch Red Cross vaccine and Heptovax B, the only one in use so far in Canada. The last is made from virus molecules obtained from the blood of carriers. However, new vaccines, grown in yeast and containing no human components, are already being tested in Toronto and American centers. Vaccine made in yeasts could be produced in large quantities and may be less expensive than obtaining antigens from carriers. Researchers foresee that as high risk groups become better protected by vaccination, their numbers will shrink and antigen donors might one day be scarce. Another kind of vaccine under development is one produced by artificial antigens, chemical look-alikes of the real thing. There's some evidence that people who become carriers lack the ability to produce one kind of antibody, and there is hope that a synthetic vaccine could persuade the immune systems of carriers to produce it. That might eliminate the carrier condition. But, at present, the vaccines in use do nothing for carriers.

Hepatitis B vaccine, devised in 1982, was slow to be accepted in North America. For one thing, it was expensive, $150 or more for the three injections into a muscle in the arm. (Injections into the buttocks were found to be less effective in stimulating production of antibodies.) But among health workers, there was another reason. Fear arose that the vaccine could be contaminated with the AIDS organism. The antigen in the vaccine was obtained largely from homosexual men, the same group most likely to have AIDS. Since then those fears have been found to be groundless. The World Health Organization has declared the vaccine safe and not a possible source of AIDS. No case of AIDS anywhere has been attributed to the vaccine.

Most countries, not surprisingly, have focused their efforts on protecting newborn babies whose mothers might be carriers. West Germany screens all mothers with tests, as are all high-risk mothers in the U.S. If the babies are given passive immunization with a globulin within 12 hours of birth and vaccinated within a week, hepatitis can be prevented in almost all babies of carriers. A large study in

Montreal, screening mothers, found that three in 1,000 pregnant women were carriers. Women most at risk of being carriers are those from parts of the world, such as China, where the disease is widespread.

Hepatitis B has been on the increase in parts of North America. In Canada, it has climbed from one case per 100,000 people in 1971 to almost 8 cases in 1985, and in Ontario even higher — to more than 12 cases per 100,000. People who get it may suffer malaise, abdominal pain, nausea, and sometimes jaundice, and typically they are off work for several weeks.

Unless you are in a high risk group, however, you need not rush out to be vaccinated. You may already have had the disease at some time without knowing it and thus have your own protection. If you are accidentally stuck with a needle when looking after a patient with hepatitis, you should be tested to determine if you are susceptible. If you are, obtain an injection of hepatitis B globulin. It's not perfect, but it is 70 per cent effective. It just might have saved the life of the Toronto surgeon had he sought globulin following the seemingly trivial, but fateful, operating room accident.

A second kind of hepatitis, called hepatitis A, was formerly called infectious hepatitis. As the name indicates, it can spread from one person to another. Patients experience fever, malaise, nausea, and sometimes jaundice; it can be a nasty illness. It develops anywhere from 15 to 50 days after contact with an infected person and is most contagious in the two weeks before jaundice appears. But unlike hepatitis B, it does not become chronic in some people, so there are no carriers. To get it from a blood transfusion is extremely rare. In North America, the number of cases is decreasing although it is still common among older children and young adults. It is also quite common in young children, especially in day-care centers, because the infection usually causes no illness in pre-schoolers and they can spread the infection without anyone being aware of the problem. Overall, type A accounts for 39 per cent of all cases of hepatitis. A vaccine against hepatitis A is not yet available.

If you or a family member has been in contact with a person with hepatitis A, you should arrange for a shot of immune globulin as soon as possible, within a maximum of two weeks. After that, it will be too late and the globulin may simply interfere with your own defenses.

It is wise to get an injection of globulin when you are traveling to underdeveloped countries, where your chances of being exposed to it are higher than at home. Some doctors also advise day-care center workers to get the protective globulin, if they are tending children still in diapers. A toddler who has been infected may shed the virus in body wastes.

Non A–non B is the awkward name for a third kind of hepatitis, the kind that most worries doctors responsible for blood banks. It can be caught from a blood transfusion but so far, unlike hepatitis B, it can't be detected in donated blood without a complicated two-step test that is not all that accurate. According to American estimates, people who receive more than three units of blood run a five to six per cent risk of developing non A–non B. Two non-specific blood tests when used together can detect the disease about one-third of the time; blood banks in the U.S. are starting to use them. But they are far from perfect and their use is controversial because many people who turn out not to have the disease show positive results. Some doctors say blood donated by such people will be wasted needlessly and the donors will be led to think, erroneously, that they are carriers of the disease. According to a recent report in the British medical journal *Lancet*, some researchers believe that after a 10-year search they have identified the virus. If they are correct, their discoveries could lead to a true test for donated blood and possibly a vaccine against it.

Hepatitis D, also known as delta hepatitis, is caused by one of the smallest microbes ever discovered. Until it was found in 1977, the cause of this kind of hepatitis was unknown. It was discovered by an Italian scientist who was investigating cells from drug users with hepatitis B. The delta virus appears to need the hepatitis B virus in order to become infective itself. It can cause acute hepatitis in hepatitis B carriers. A test to detect it is expected to be commercially available soon. The vaccine that prevents hepatitis B protects against it by depriving it of its essential partner.

INFLUENZA

"I think I've got a touch of the flu." Probably most of us have said that at one time or another when we're feeling a bit under the weather. But as anybody who has had a full-blown bout of influenza well knows, you don't get touched by flu, you get steam-rollered. Your throat is sore, you have a bone-shaking cough, you ache everywhere, and you're feverish, drenching the sheets with sweat at one time, shivering with chills at another. There are two major kinds of flu bugs that doctors call Type A and Type B. Periodically cases of flu sweep across the continent like a gigantic tidal wave. After World War I, in 1918, soldiers brought home to Canada a flu virus that had already been causing epidemics in other parts of the world. But it was a bug new to eight million Canadians, the population of the country at that time. Virtually everybody was susceptible and the illness swept through community after community, from east to west. Within two or three months it had taken almost 50,000 lives, nearly as many lives as Canada lost in combat during the four-year war.

Around the world, that pandemic of 1918 is estimated to have killed between 20 and 22 million people in just a few months, many of them healthy, young adults, not ordinarily the segment of a population in which flu is deadly. It was known as Spanish influenza. By the fall of 1918, it had been caught by one of every six Canadians. It was first reported in the United States in March 1918 by American servicemen stationed in Kansas. Within five weeks, more than 1,200 soldiers at the base had been stricken.

An outbreak of disease that spreads through a whole population is called a pandemic, literally a huge epidemic. In recent years, flu has been so widespread as to be termed a pandemic on two occasions, 1957 and 1968. More than a quarter of North Americans were affected in each of those years, and lesser outbreaks, called epidemics, have occurred 17 times. An epidemic has been estimated to cost the continent more than $1-billion in medical care and time lost from work. But more distressing than the financial loss is the increase in deaths among people over the age of 65, who succumb to the flu itself or pneumonia that often develops in the frail, or among people with chronic heart, lung, or kidney disease.

Vaccination against flu every year is strongly recommended for the elderly and for others at high risk because of underlying diseases.

The problem with flu is that having it once doesn't mean you are protected forever. The Type A virus is a sneaky devil that can change itself and appear in a new disguise so your immune system doesn't recognize it again after a first encounter. Type A has two antigens, proteins that tip off the immune cells that the virus is present and which stimulate them to begin antibody production. But those antigens are altered every so often. If you had, say, Hong Kong flu, one variety of Type A, you'd be protected against that strain, but the next flu bug to come around might be Philippine flu. Its antigens are different and would not be instantly recognized by your body. Flu types are commonly named after the place they are first identified.

Researchers believe Type A viruses undergo such changes in other species. They particularly suspect it happens in birds. Genes in the virus instruct it how to make antigens. Scientists think a Type A virus infects a bird and exchanges genetic material with a bird virus. The result is a flu virus with new antigens.

Every year public health scientists and drug companies that produce vaccines try to predict which strains of flu are likely to be most common in the coming fall and winter, the peak flu period. New strains typically are first seen in the southern hemisphere, providing some advance warning for the next season in the northern hemisphere. The prediction is usually made about February and vaccine manufacturers then begin intense work, developing and producing the right vaccine for fall.

Type B flu is not quite as tricky as its fellow troublemaker. It is more stable and undergoes fewer antigen alterations. Nevertheless, it too can change, and flu vaccine may contain protection against different kinds of B from year to year. Flu vaccine has been available since 1963. But, at the same time, the numbers of people at greatest risk of complications from flu keep increasing. More people are living into their 70s and 80s. Improved medical care is extending the lifespan of people with chronic diseases, with transplanted organs, or with conditions of the immune system that make them vulnerable to infections. While the vaccines, made with killed viruses, are highly effective in stimulating antibody production in healthy adults, those who most need the protection are often less able to respond to the vaccine. In such people, even if a vaccine can't protect them fully against a flu bug, it does prevent complications, such as pneumonia. There is a possibility that giving flu vaccine to elderly people by mouth, rather than by injection into muscle, may be more effective. At Queen's University in Kingston, Ontario, researchers have found that, at least in animals, immune responses in the intestine remain vigorous into old age, although other parts of the immune network become less efficient.

In general, these people are recommended for vaccinations against flu:

- Adults and children over six months with heart or lung disorders severe enough that they were required to have medical care or be admitted to hospital in the past year — in particular, children with cystic fibrosis, severe chronic asthma, and congenital heart disease.
- Residents of any age in nursing homes or long-stay hospitals.
- Health care workers who have extensive contact with high-risk groups, and who might therefore transmit flu germs to their vulnerable patients.
- People over 65.
- Adults and children with diabetes, kidney diseases, or immune suppression (for any reason).
- People who provide essential community services, such as firefighters and police, not because they are at higher risk of flu but because they are needed on the job.

Vaccinations can be given when it becomes evident to public health doctors that a flu virus is spreading in the community. But it takes two to three weeks for your immune system to build up its defenses and you can be susceptible during that time. People who should not be vaccinated are those who have severe allergic reactions to eggs. Eggs are used to grow the viruses for vaccine production. Pregnant women should wait until after the first three months, just to be on the safe side, although no hazards to the fetus have been seen. People running fevers should wait until their symptoms of illness have disappeared.

In many laboratories researchers continue to search for ways to outwit the wily Type A bug and make a vaccine that would work against all Type As. One promising finding is a protein produced by all As which appears to be responsible for attracting T cells to the site of infection. This newly discovered antigen, shared by all As, was discovered by researchers at Northwestern University, Evanston, Illinois. The discovery has brought hope of a more permanent vaccine that remains effective even when Type A viruses shift genes.

Researchers are also investigating new ways to give vaccines. In Britain, a preparation sprayed into the nose is being tested against two kinds of flu bugs. The idea is that virus, put into the nose, will cause antibodies to be produced against it right in the nasal passages. But the virus, although it is alive, has been treated so that it can't stand body heat. Once it leaves the relatively cool passages of the nose, on its way to sites deeper in the body, it dies. It is unable to start up an infection elsewhere.

PNEUMONIA

People who get flu, especially the elderly, are prone to pneumonia caused by bacteria. The bacteria take advantage of the fact that body defenses have been weakened by the flu virus. Virtually all the same people considered to be in high risk groups for flu are also considered to be vulnerable to bacterial pneumonia, whether or not they catch flu. Pneumonia is still a leading cause of death in North America, taking some 60,000 lives a year. It starts with sudden shaking chills and a sharp pain in the chest, a high fever, headache, and lung congestion. Bouts of painful coughing occur with production of copious amounts of sputum, at first pinkish in color but later becoming rusty or yellow as the crisis is passed.

In otherwise healthy people, white blood cells, plentiful in lung tissues, set up their lines of defense. The cells known as phagocytes surround and gobble up the invading micro-organisms; B cells produce antibodies; and T helper cells orchestrate the counter-attack. About half of all cases of pneumonia are caused by bacteria. Of these cases, the majority are the result of infections by bacteria called pneumococci. In its virulent form, the pneumococcus produces a coat or capsule forming an envelope around pairs of bacterial cells. Capsules are formed of a variety of carbohydrates, called polysaccharides, and each can be recognized by the immune system, setting off a warning of an enemy invasion. Scientists make use of the variety of carbohydrates on the bacteria capsules to create vaccines. One produced in 1977 contained 14 polysaccharides. A newer one developed in 1983 contains 23. That gives the immune system a pretty good chance of being ready for a pneumoccocus should it appear. More than eight out of 10 times, the bug will be in a capsule containing one of those 23 antigens, and so the immune system will recognize it as an enemy.

Doctors recommend pneumonia vaccination for virtually the same groups of people for whom they advise flu vaccine (see above). Recent studies have shown that the two vaccines can be given safely at the same time. Pneumonia vaccine, however, should be given only once. In fact, it's been learned that a second shot, or booster, can cause adverse effects. It is not recommended for healthy pregnant women because its safety during pregnancy has not been evaluated.

It was once believed that when antibiotics, so effective against bacteria, were developed, bacterial pneumonia would no longer be life-threatening. The false sense of safety may have slowed research into vaccines, postponing their development. But recently, penicillin-resistant strains of pneumococci have been discovered, first appearing in South Africa. Not only penicillin, but almost all antibiotics, are ineffective against them, and the U.S. National Foundation for Infectious Diseases has stressed that this alarming discovery makes vaccination more important than ever.

RABIES

In the summer of 1985, a special occasion was marked by the medical profession: the centennial of the modern era of immunization. On July 6, 1885, French chemist Louis Pasteur and his colleagues injected the first of 14 daily doses of a material into a nine-year-old boy named Joseph Meister who had been bitten two days earlier by a rabid dog.

For four years, Pasteur had been conducting intensive research trying to make a vaccine. He'd put the rabies virus into rabbits' spinal cords to obtain a weakened version of the virus and he'd tested it on animals with success. Still, this was a child, and the decision to try the vaccine was not easy to make. "The child's death seemed inevitable. I decided, not without acute and harrowing anxiety, as may be imagined, to apply to Joseph Meister the method which I had found consistently successful with dogs," he wrote later.

It worked, saving the child's life. Within a short time the procedure had been widely adopted and rabies treatment centers were set up from Warsaw to New York, and from Budapest to Shanghai. But what Pasteur had done was to have far wider implications than simply treatment for rabies. He had proven that infectious diseases, caused by viruses that could not even be seen, could be cured or prevented if scientists learned how to work with the immune system. He showed viruses could be manipulated and weakened to make them safe, and that immunity could be brought about without danger to people's health.

Rabies is one of the oldest diseases known to man. Over thousands of years, a cry of alarm of "mad dog" brought terror to the heart. Those who became ill with rabies invariably died. Fortunately, humans are not very susceptible to the rabies virus; many who are bitten by rabid animals don't develop it. Between 1925 and 1985, only 21 cases were recorded in humans in Canada, although the country has a large number of rabid animals. The first case recorded was the death, in 1819, of the Duke of Richmond, then governor-in-chief of Canada, who was bitten either by a pet fox or his dog while he traveled from Kingston, Ontario, to Quebec City. By the mid-1950s, the province of Ontario had gained the unwanted title of "rabies capital of North America" as red foxes and skunks became infected and spread the disease.

Once commonly called hydrophobia, rabies is caused by a rhabdovirus that is carried in the salivary glands of animals. When a person is bitten, the rhabdovirus gets into the wound, traveling to nerves where it hides and multiplies for two to seven weeks. Then symptoms — drowsiness, loss of appetite, and fever — appear. Fluids cause spasms of the throat so the person won't drink. As the central nervous system and brain become involved, the victim alternately acts wildly or lethargically and dies of vascular collapse and respiratory failure.

With the Pasteur vaccine, death rates dropped substantially in the world. But because it was made with rabbit tissue, some people had adverse reactions affecting the nervous system. While your immune system rejects cells from other people, it reacts even more violently against molecules from other species. New modifications of Pasteur's vaccine were developed, made in chicks and in duck eggs, which were less likely to cause adverse reactions. Yet, people still had to endure many painful injections, and some had allergic responses to eggs, risking complications.

With the 1950s came a breakthrough. Dr. Leonard Hayflick found special cells in human fetal tissue, called diploid cells, that would grow unchanged in the laboratory. Viruses could be grown in them instead of in animals or poultry eggs. For the first time, a vaccine could be made that did not carry a risk of severe complications. Called human diploid cell vaccine, it could be used not only after exposure to a rabid animal but also as a preventive measure to vaccinate veterinarians and other animal handlers at higher than average risk. Virus particles in the vaccine cause the production of antibodies in the body within seven to 10 days. At the same time as the first injection is given to a bitten or scratched person, rabies immune globulin, containing antibodies to rabies, is injected to provide the person with protection until his or her own immune system begins producing its own antibodies. The globulin comes from the blood of people who have already been vaccinated and so have antibodies that can be harvested.

Since 1980, when the diploid cell vaccine became available in Canada, there has been only one report of a failure among the 1,000 to 3,000 people treated each year. In that one case, the rabies globulin was not given along with the vaccine. The last victim, before the vaccine was available, was a little Ontario girl bitten by the family cat. Nation-wide, nine of every 100,000 people received anti-rabies treatment between 1979 and 1983; in Ontario the rate was 22.7 per 100,000.

If you or a family member is bitten by an animal, domestic or wild, that might be rabid, the most important thing to do is immediately to wash the wound thoroughly with soap or detergent and water, or water alone if no soap is available. Public health authorities say immediate washing is probably the most effective method of prevention. Afterwards, apply alcohol or iodine and see your doctor. If possible, the wound should not be sutured.

Your local public health department will tell you what is to be done about determining whether the animal is rabid. If it is a family pet that is not obviously ill, it may be kept under observation by a veterinarian for 10 days. If it remains well for that time, rabies is unlikely and your pet may not have to be destroyed.

Some parts of the world are rabies free. Great Britain is one such place and keeps the disease out by constant vigilance and quarantine of all animals coming in from other countries. In North America, widespread vaccination of family dogs is helping to curb the disease, and in some regions, ingenious programs have been developed for getting vaccine to wild animals. In Ontario, for example, vaccine is put in pouches and tucked inside meatballs, scattered in the wilderness. One day, with a concerted effort, rabies may be under control throughout the world.

VACCINES FOR TRAVELERS

In 1985, excitement was high among researchers concerned with some major killer and crippler diseases that afflict millions of people in the world. Before the age of jet travel, they were not of urgent concern to most North Americans. But that's far from the situation today. There is an abundance of travelers who may need protection from infectious diseases they would not encounter at home. The research was good news to them, because, for the first time, scientists were announcing the development of vaccines that held high promise of preventing malaria, cholera, and leprosy. It may be some time before they are fully tested and widely available. But at last research is on track, discovering enough about the infective organisms to indicate that vaccines are possible.

Malaria

Malaria affects more than 200 to 400 million people, most of them living in a wide tropical band that stretches around the world. For a short time in the 1960s, we foolishly believed the disease could be conquered with pesticides to wipe out the mosquitoes that spread the disease to man. Malaria is caused by parasites that use mosquitoes as airplanes in which to ride and the stingers of the insects as needles with which to inject themselves into people. Our optimism was premature. We had underestimated the enemy. The parasites and the mosquitoes adapted, becoming resistant to DDT and other insecticides, and within 20 years there was a resurgence of malaria. In Africa, it is a major cause of death in children, in some regions killing up to half its victims.

The two worst species of the parasite, which is called Plasmodium, are Plasmodium falciparum and Plasmodium vivax. They are one-celled organisms that change shape and form, much as caterpillars turn into butterflies, during the course of their development. The first stage, spear-shaped and called sporozoite, lives in the mosquitoes' salivary glands and gets into a person's bloodstream when the mosquito bites to get a blood dinner. Some 60 kinds of mosquito can carry the parasite. The first type of malaria vaccine devised was aimed at the sporozoite and was made possible when New York University scientists discovered a protein on the sporozoite against which antibodies are formed.

In the human body, there is little time to produce antibodies when a sporozoite is inserted by a mosquito. Within an hour, each sporozoite makes its way to a liver cell. The liver cell is then sentenced to forced labor. One sporozoite can turn a liver cell into a factory that produces 5,000 to 10,000 parasites. But the parasites have a different shape from the sporozoites. Instead of being spear-shaped, they are tiny spheres. The immune system can no longer recognize them as the same problem. There is no rapid defense.

The round parasites are called merozoites, and they head off from their liver cell incubators to take up residence in red blood cells, where they reproduce themselves until the cell bursts, spilling out 10 or 20 more merozoites ready to take over more red cells. It's the bursting of red cells that causes the chills and fever of malaria. A merozoite has molecular "jaws" that take hold of the red cell so the parasite can force entry. A second malaria vaccine may be developed against these jaws. New York scientists have been able to make thousands of copies of the jaws, in a process called cloning. Put into a vaccine preparation, they stimulate the human body to make antibodies against them.

In the ordinary course of malaria infection, the merozoite, like the sporozoite, is only free in the bloodstream — where it's likely to be spotted by the immune system — for a short time. There's little chance for attack before it is gone. Furthermore, researchers have found the parasite is able to sucker the immune system, by producing plenty of decoy antigens on its coat that antibodies go after. The parasite then slips out of its fuzzy coat and hustles off to hide in a cell.

But the two vaccines may be able to give the crafty organism a one-two punch. Immune cells will be primed to recognize the name-badge of the sporozoite, and if some of those escape detection and produce merozoites, then their jaws, already familiar to body defenders, will set off another line of attack.

In Canada in 1980, about 600 people were reported to have malaria. Until 1984, the number of cases had declined, but then began rising again, an increase Health and Welfare Canada attributed to a resurgence of the disease in South America and other tropical countries visited by Canadians. In Great Britain the number of cases rose from 100 in 1970 to 1,472 in 1982. In the U.S. malaria infections among travelers rose almost sevenfold between 1973 and 1983. Until the vaccines become available, travelers are advised to protect themselves with weekly doses of a drug called chloroquine if they are visiting regions where malaria is widespread. The drug is not a guarantee that you won't get malaria, however, and in some areas, chloroquine-resistant parasites have been found. Symptoms can develop as early as eight days after infection, or not until months later, but need prompt medical attention.

Cholera

Cholera is said to be no stranger in North America, yet today we don't think of it as a big problem. It is still widespread in East Africa, where it kills 100,000 people a year. That number increased in 1985 because of drought that caused a water shortage and contaminated water supplies. Cholera organisms, taken into the body in water, pass quickly through the stomach and thrive in the intestines causing the primary symptoms of the disease, severe diarrhea and dehydration. It's also common in the Middle East and parts of Europe. But international health regulations no longer require proof of vaccination against the disease for visitors to foreign lands. The main reason is that the vaccine we had for many years really wasn't much good. In addition, the risk to travelers was quite low. However, some countries still demand proof of vaccination. But travelers are often provided with exception certificates, rather than proof of vaccination, in order to satisfy requirements of those countries.

Recently, in Adelaide, Australia, scientists devised a vaccine that is taken by mouth. They say it works more directly, producing antibodies in the digestive tract and preventing the cholera bacteria from producing toxin. Produced by genetic engineering techniques, through which germs that cause cholera are produced by bacteria, providing a plentiful supply with which to make the vaccine, it enables the immune system to be on the alert in advance of naturally acquired infection. One of its developers has said that it will probably take until 1989 before its safety and effectiveness can be proven, but the outcome looks extremely hopeful.

Leprosy

For many years scientists had been searching for some way to make a vaccine against leprosy, but it seemed futile. No matter how hard they tried, the leprosy bacillus defied all attempts to grow it in the laboratory. But in the 1970s, researchers acquired an unexpected assistant: the armadillo. The scaly little creature could do exactly what they needed: grow large quantities of the organism, in effect acting like a living test tube for the researchers. It turned the dream of a vaccine into a reasonable hope.

Leprosy, also called Hansen's disease, isn't highly contagious. Only people in long-term contact with patients are at risk. Yet throughout the ages, in every culture, leprosy has evoked horror and fear. People with the disease were shunned and isolated from society. A few cases are diagnosed in Canada each year, but the disease is mainly found in Africa, Asia, and Latin America, where it affects nearly 11 million people. Yet, until the armadillo came along, research into prevention had lagged behind research into other diseases. Few scientists had any expertise in leprosy research. But in 1975, some specialists, along with others in immunology, began a remarkable international program. Leprosy bacilli were harvested from patients in India and South America and shipped to Louisiana in the U.S. where they were injected into armadillos. Armadillo tissues were sent to London, England, where a group of researchers were expert at separating the bacilli from tissue. The purified bacilli were then sent to Sweden and Norway, where still other scientists analyzed them for antigens, the molecules that could cause antibodies to be produced against them.

From there, the bacilli were shipped to New York and Atlanta, Georgia, to test the effectiveness of the antigens in guinea pigs and mice as stimulators of protective antibodies. A bank was set up to store bacilli, antigens, and genes of the bacilli so they could be shared and distributed to researchers all over the world. And now three candidate vaccines — two from India, one from Caracus — have come off the drawing board and are undergoing testing. Dr. Barry Bloom of New York, chairman of the program steering committee, has said, "It is always easier to seek funds for drugs to treat illness than it is for supporting research to develop vaccines that will perhaps prevent disease. It may be worth mentioning that 12 years of operations and research for the eradication of smallpox cost approximately $46-million and that the United States saves $500-million each year in not having to vaccinate overseas travelers." Dr. Bloom adds that if these leprosy vaccines, or second generation versions of them, live up to their promise, it would be possible to eliminate leprosy from the face of the earth as it was smallpox.

Yellow Fever

Currently the only kind of vaccination you might be required to have before you travel to certain parts of the world is against yellow fever. The disease is caused by a virus that might infect you if you are bitten by a mosquito common in the tropics. Jungle yellow fever is a disease of monkeys in Africa and Central and South America that is transmitted to man by mosquitoes. Travelers, or people such as oil company and forestry workers, living in parts of the world where there is yellow fever, should get a single shot of the live-virus vaccine. It is available only at yellow fever vaccination centers approved by the World Health Organization. In Canada and the U.S., the address of your nearest center may be obtained from your local public health department.

Prevention

Until vaccines against malaria and cholera become widely available, there are some protective steps you can take. In malaria, areas, avoid contact with mosquitoes by remaining in well-screened areas between dusk and dawn; use mosquito nets and wear clothes that cover most of the body. Take insect repellent with you and keep exposed parts of the body sprayed. Cholera is caused by a species of bacteria that lives in water, including the Gulf Coast in the U.S. and brackish inland lakes, and can infect shellfish. It is possible, therefore to get cholera from eating raw oysters or undercooked crab and by swimming in infected waters. The risk, however, is low in North America, and ordinarily doctors only warn people with liver disease to avoid these hazards entirely. The risk of complications and possible death from cirrhosis of the liver for people whose livers are already damaged, is substantial.

People with leprosy are no danger to travelers. As mentioned, the disease, which today is usually called Hansen's disease to avoid the stigma deeply ingrained in the name leprosy, is spread from person to person only after prolonged contact. It is not spread by insects or water.

NEW VACCINES

Already here, or on the way soon, are a number of vaccines to protect children and young adults. Among them is one that will save the lives of many babies who would otherwise succumb to meningitis. Another one, which will shortly be ready, will help young North Americans avoid a common, strength-sapping ailment, infectious mononucleosis. But more important, it may also be able to prevent two kinds of cancer in other parts of the world. There is a third new vaccine on the way that may make visits to the dentist a lot easier (see below).

Meningitis

In 1985, the first vaccine to be released for public use in North America since 1969, came on the market. It was devised to protect against a bacterial infection that is a prime cause of meningitis in babies. The bacterium is called Hemophilus influenzae type B, or Hib for short, and it causes as many infections today as the polio virus once did before we had polio vaccines. The most common complication is meningitis, an inflammation of the membrane covering the brain.

The Canadian Pediatric Society and the American Academy of Pediatrics have recommended that all children receive the one-shot vaccine at the age of two. It can be given as early as 18 months if the child will be attending a day-care center, or up to the sixth birthday if it hasn't been given earlier. A study in Finland of some 50,000 children given the vaccine in 1974 when they were ages three months to five years, found that it gave good protection to those 24 months of age or older. Before that their immune systems were not mature enough to respond, and even at 18 months some might need a second shot later.

Hib vaccine would be even more useful if it could be given to babies under the age of two. Sixty per cent of meningitis cases are in children under the age of 18 months. With that in mind, researchers at Connaught Laboratories in Toronto, Canada, in 1986, announced that they are devising a vaccine which they believe will work in infants. It involves a new kind of technology called carrier-hapten technology, developed by Dr. Lance Gordon, a Connaught senior research scientist.

The vaccine that works in older children doesn't work in babies because until about the age of two children's B-cell system — the line of defense that produces antibodies — isn't fully developed. Ordinarily, bacterial infections are handled by B cells, rather than T cells, the other defense army. The new technology brings T cells into the fight. Using a chemical called a hapten as a carrier, the Toronto scientists attached to it a Hib molecule (antigen) and a molecule of diphtheria toxin. Babies are vaccinated against diphtheria in the first year and have immune cells that recognize the toxin. When T cells of a baby who has been vaccinated against it zero in on toxin antigen, they discover the Hib antigen and order B cells to make antibodies against it. Early studies show that babies, given three doses of vaccine at two, four and six months of age, make high levels of protective antibodies against Hemophilus bacteria. Further research and testing for safety of the Connaught vaccine is underway.

There are an estimated 30,000 cases of Hib a year in North America. Hib causes approximately half of all cases of meningitis. Meningitis can, in some cases, be fatal. In about a third of cases, it leaves some permanent nervous system damage. Its symptoms include a severe headache and a stiff and painful neck. The chance of a child's getting a Hib infection in the first five years of life is calculated to be one in 200. The bacterium can cause a number of other illnesses, including pneumonia and inflammation of the heart covering called pericarditis.

Mononucleosis

Sometimes called the kissing disease, or mono, infectious mononucleosis is a viral disease that commonly spreads in adolescents or college students, causing fever, a general run-down feeling, tonsilitis, enlarged spleen, and sometimes a rash of tiny red spots. In their blood are white cells, lymphocytes, that look abnormal. The organism that causes it is the Epstein-Barr virus. Vaccines against the virus are under development in Chicago and Bristol, England, and at the University of Saskatchewan, Canada.

The exciting possibility of such a vaccine is that it might be able to help prevent two kinds of cancer: Burkitt's lymphoma, which occurs in African children, and naso-pharyngeal carcinoma, common in the Orient. The E-B virus has been linked to those cancers and is probably a co-factor with some other cancer agent in those populations. The virus, a member of the herpes family, gets into antibody-producing B cells. In North America, most people who become infected are able to mount an effective immune response and become protected against catching the bug again. In AIDS patients, whose immune systems have been demolished, the E-B virus can cause cancer of B cells; the cells multiply wildly and develop a Burkitt's-like lymphoma. Doctors say the role of the virus as a cause of lymphoma in immune-suppressed people becomes increasingly evident as they study AIDS patients, patients with liver and bone marrow transplants, and people in Africa with Burkitt's lymphoma. A vaccine, therefore, would have much greater value than just as a prevention of kissing disease. In Chicago, an animal vaccine has been developed that protects monkeys from E-B infections, and also from cancers (lymphomas) the animals get as a result of the infection. And in England, Dr. M.A. Epstein, one of the discovers of the virus bearing his name, has devised another animal vaccine in marmosets. The animal vaccines are models from which to learn and are not intended for use in people. But they have shown that vaccination against the virus is possible.

Strep Throat

Sore throats are almost as common as icicles in Canada in winter, and about one in every 10 of them is caused by bacteria, primarily members of the streptococcus family. Before there were antibiotics to treat strep throat, many people developed serious complications, including rheumatic fever, rheumatic heart disease, and inflammation of the kidneys. Until recently, scientists searching for ways to make a strep vaccine had been stumped. There are about 80 strains of the bacteria and a vaccine against one strain would be unlikely to protect against another.

However, a short time ago, researchers in Minnesota

found a key to the puzzle. They identified a gene in the bacterium that controls the bug's on and off switch. When the switch is on, the organism is able to fend off an attack by immune cells by producing proteins attached to its outer surface that fool the immune system. At the same time, a carboyhydrate and an enzyme are produced that increase the bacterium's virulence. The researchers found that by taking away genetic material, they could deprive the bacterium of all three of its weapons. In effect, they turned the bacterium's own protein weapon against the bacterium itself. In a vaccine they show it to the immune system for what it is, so immune cells are no longer fooled. To do this, scientists copy the gene that orders production of the protein weapon and use it to make a supply of the protein. They combine proteins of different strains into one vaccine because each strain of strep bug makes a different protein. Presented to the immune system by means of the vaccine, the proteins each arouse an antibody response. The immune system remembers and the next time any variety of strep germ tries to produce its protein weapon, it will be recognized as an enemy and vigorously attacked. If the vaccine lives up to its promise, strep throat could become a disease of the past.

Tooth Decay

The day may be coming soon when children will go to the dentist to be immunized against cavities. Dental researchers in the United States and in France are developing protection against the bacteria responsible for tooth decay. Bacteria, which are members of the strep family, called Streptococci mutans, accumulate around the teeth and stick to them, converting sugar into acids that can dissolve tooth enamel, letting decay and cavities begin. The organisms use a protein to hang onto teeth so tightly that tooth-brushing can't budge the pests. At Washington University in St. Louis, Missouri, researchers are using the protein in a vaccine. Antibodies are produced against it. And without their "glue" the bacteria can't adhere to teeth. They drift around harmlessly.

The American team expects that the vaccine will be made as a pill to be given to children as soon as baby teeth appear. In France, researchers are using the same bacterium, but injecting it; the vaccine reduced cavities by 60 to 80 per cent in monkeys, also susceptible to tooth decay. However, both groups must yet prove beyond any question of doubt that the bits of bacterial protein they use as antigens to stimulate antibody production cannot themselves cause disease, and it will be some time yet before all the checks for safety are completed.

NEW BREEDS OF VACCINES

A small revolution in vaccines has been taking place in research laboratories in recent years. While we've been fussing about safety of vaccines long in use, such as the whooping cough vaccine, many scientists have taken off in directions never before traveled in vaccine research. They're coming up with possibilities that will astound us.

Since the time of Edward Jenner two centuries ago, it has always been thought essential that a vaccine contain the germ, or part of it, that it is designed to protect against. We know our immune cells must meet up with an invasive organism before they can prepare a defense, and we know memory immune cells remember previous invaders and are ready for them next time around. But now scientists are saying there are ways to make vaccines without using any part of a microbe.

In North America and Europe, this whole new ballgame of vaccines is being played hard and fast because it means a wide array of new vaccines may be possible, perhaps even some against cancer, and that tomorrow's vaccines will be the safest and most effective ever seen.

What kind of molecular magic does it take to make a vaccine containing no part of a virus, bacteria, or parasite?

The trick, say the researchers, is to make fake antigens in the laboratory. Antigens are particles that the immune system recognizes. Antibodies, with claws that fit an antigen snugly, latch onto it. The surprising part is that these phony antigens are actually antibodies themselves. But they spur immune cells to make real antibodies against the germ.

Now wait a minute! How can an antibody be an antigen? Scientists have taught us that an antigen and its antibody fit together like a lock and key. The antibody and antigen are, structurally, the exact reverse images of each other. But suppose you took an antibody and considered it as an antigen. For example, if you took a human antibody and put it into another species, the animals's immune system would see it as a foreign invader and make antibodies. So the scientists take an antigen from a microbe and produce antibodies to it in the laboratory. Then they scoop up those antibodies, inject them into mice, where they are antigens to the mouse and the immune cells of the mice make antibodies against the antibodies. This new round of antibodies is the reverse picture of the first antibodies. That, of course, makes them the same shape as the germ antigens. Presto! The researchers have a particle that is just like the germ in shape but does not cause disease. Although it looks the same, it is chemically different. But the immune system doesn't care about the chemistry. It looks like an enemy, so immune cells react as if it is an enemy.

To put it simplistically, if A is a mirror image of B and B is a mirror image of C, then A and C must be the same. If you wanted the immune system to make antibodies against A, you could show it C instead of A. The antibodies to A and C would be the same. Or, as one scientist puts it, "Consider the germ a key. We make a wax impression of the key and from that make a forgery of the real key. It's made out of different material but it still fits the lock. It's a safe forgery because it isn't a germ that causes disease."

(Still with me? It is rather heavy going. But for those who are determined to slog on, there is a bit more to understand. The rest of you are excused and may go get a cup of tea.) Your immune system, in the ordinary course of events, makes antibodies against its own antibodies. It is one method it uses to regulate the supply of antibodies in the body. More than 10 years ago, an interacting antibody network was proposed by Niels Jerne of the Basel Institute of Immunology, Switzerland, who shared the Nobel prize in 1984 for his work.

An antibody has, as might be expected, one part that determines which antigen it matches. Each antibody, remember, fits one specific antigen and no other. Scientists call this part the idiotype, meaning loosely "one's own thing." But when high levels of antibodies with one kind of idiotype are reached, a control mechanism comes into play.

In effect the "thermostat" is turned down. Other antibodies, called anti-idiotype antibodies, are formed against the first antibodies to keep control of the process. There would be no sense in having your body chock-a-block with antibodies that fought only measles. After you've recovered from say, measles, those antibodies fade away, leaving only a few on guard in case of a repeat encounter. They disappear because they are taken out of action by anti-idiotypes. It explains how the immune system rises to the occasion when needed and then slumps back into inactivity after the battle. Dr. Jerne said that the immune system is constantly trying to keep itself balanced. Every time a battle disturbs its equilibrium, mechanisms, including anti-antibodies and suppressor cells, are called on to put it back on an even keel.

Taking their cue from the immune system's own ingenious techniques, some researchers are using similar strategy in attempts to develop vaccines against AIDS and cancers. Nobody would risk using the real virus that causes AIDS in making a vaccine. But there are hopes that one day it will be possible to devise a vaccine made with fraud virus particles, safe and non-infective. It will take time and intensive laboratory work.

Vaccines against cancers pose a slightly different dilemma. Scientists have had little luck discovering antigens specific to tumor cells. But, says one top researcher, scientists can't find the antigens, but the immune system can. "It's like a police force with well-trained bloodhounds. The immune system can sniff out antigens." To give the "bloodhounds" the scent, cancer scientists in Buffalo have put cancer cells into mice. The mice make antibodies to them. The scientists collect the antibodies and grow them in vast quantities in the laboratory. On those antibodies are the segments (idiotypes) that are mirror images of cancer cell antigens. But the scientists want to create artificial antigens that look just like cancer cell antigens. To do that they put the first antibodies they made into other mice, which make antibodies against them. This second generation of antibodies looks the same as cancer antigens. Who said understanding molecular biology is easy?

So far so good. But at that point the research magicians must perform another trick. They must get the "mouseness" out of the preparation. Otherwise, if such a vaccine were put into a human, the person's immune system would react strongly against antigens identifying "mouse." As we know, our bodies vehemently reject anything from a non-human species. As soon as immune cells saw "mouse," their reaction would destroy the vaccine before there was any chance of its working. The scientists have figured out ways to remove the mouse genes and replace them with human genes, but they have a long way to go before such cancer vaccines are a reality.

However, the fake antigen technique has been used by French scientists to make the first anti-body vaccine. It is designed to protect against a worm that causes schistosomiasis, also called river disease, which next to malaria is mankind's worst parasite disease. In other research centers, studies are aimed at producing these kinds of vaccines against flu, rabies, hepatitis, and strep infections.

In other approaches to making new or better vaccines, researchers are using genetic engineering. A whole virus causes disease but the antigens on the virus will not. Scientists have learned how to make viral antigens without the rest of the virus. They take virus genes that carry the instructions for making virus antigens and insert them into the genetic material of yeast. The yeast obligingly produces lots of the antigen to be used in a vaccine. One possible development with this technique is a vaccine against herpes.

More startling is the possibility of inserting these virus antigen genes into the cowpox virus contained in smallpox vaccine. Scientists say this virus has plenty of room for extra genes and could accommodate 15 or 20 from other germs. That might mean one shot could protect against a broad spectrum of diseases. When the vaccine is injected into a person, the immune system would, henceforth, recognize not only cowpox but also the other germs whose antigens it is shown.

Not all scientists think it is wise to fiddle with smallpox vaccine to turn it into a carrier of other germ antigens. They're fearful that the manipulation might alter the cowpox virus in an unknown and dangerous way. Much remains to be learned before this technique could be considered safe.

Yet another new pathway to vaccines is to make chemical copies of short pieces of virus called peptides. The copies contain no biological or living material, but antibodies are formed against them. The vaccines could be taken in pills. The method was first used to create a vaccine to protect cattle against foot and mouth disease. French and Israeli scientists have developed the first one for human use. It's a diphtheria vaccine that they predict will be cheaper than diphtheria toxoid.

Still other research groups are figuring out how to outsmart flu viruses. The bugs are able to change readily, every so often, because instead of having their genes strung like beads on one long strand like most germs, they have eight separate genes that they can swap around. That seemed to make a vaccine impossible. But now, scientists are capitalizing on the separate gene structure to swap, deliberately, genes from one kind of flu bug to another. With the right combinations of genes, they produce a hybrid that doesn't cause illness.

One vaccine made that way was first tested in England, in 1984. Fourteen volunteers were given it by means of nose drops, the nose being the route by which flu viruses ordinarily get into the body. Doctors theorized that immune battle lines would be formed in the nasal passage and upper respiratory tract and that the vaccine would work better given nasally than by injection. Early results prove them right. Development of the vaccine continues.

What about that persistent nuisance, the old-fashioned common cold? It is caused by so many different kinds of viruses that vaccines may never be the pathway to protection. But nasal sprays of interferons, substances the body itself produces when viruses infect cells, are already being tested. American and Australian researchers have found that one spray, containing alpha interferon, was effective against 40 per cent of colds — those caused by germs called rhinoviruses — but not against other kinds of cold viruses. Such sprays may be available by prescription before too long.

But there is some hope the dozens, perhaps hundreds, of cold viruses may have one thing in common that might make possible a one-shot cure. American researchers have recently shown that a cold virus is a 20-sided sphere. In each sphere is a cleft or dimple. Scientists think the receptors by which a virus locks to a cell that it is going to invade may be in those clefts, which are too narrow to be entered by antibodies.

If their theory is correct, molecules tiny enough to enter could be devised; they would block the site, preventing a virus from hooking onto a cell and therefore preventing infection. The tiny blocking molecules would be carried by laboratory-made antibodies specially designed to track down cold viruses.

Many health care experts say that the exciting potential for new vaccines has come at the right time. Society, worried about ever-increasing costs of medical treatment, is much more interested in prevention of disease today. As some have said, in North America the focus has been only on disease, not on keeping people well. Our so-called health care system has really been a sick-care system. In future, vaccines may help turn that around.

CHAPTER 12

A Glimpse Into Tomorrow

When Sally Ride, America's first woman in space, soared aloft on the space shuttle, she had in her care equipment to produce a valuable hormone. The experiment marks the beginning of a potential space industry: the manufacture of drugs is expected to be one of the first businesses to be established beyond earth's bounds. There are plans for full scale manufacturing of at least one product on unmanned space platforms in the 1990s. The tragic explosion in January 1986 of the Challenger space shuttle, which killed seven astronauts, has delayed space projects; how soon pharmaceutical products will be produced remains to be seen. But there's little doubt that space drugs will be a wave of the future. In orbit, in zero gravity, it is possible to produce substances in a purer form than can be achieved on earth. Miniscule capsules, to encase pancreatic cells for transplants, are more perfectly round (a desirable shape for acceptance in the body) when produced in a low gravity environment. Immune system products are almost certain to be produced there.

Other studies in space have delved into the effects of gravity on immune cells and microscopic organisms. German scientists, for example, sent millions of bacterial spores on a 10-day orbit via the shuttle Columbia, to learn more about how changes occur in living cells as their environment is altered. European studies have also found that in zero gravity, lymphocytes multiplied far less than usual. Investigation of white cells of four astronauts showed that they were able to produce antibodies as efficiently as ever. Yet there is an indication that the white blood cells of space-travelers lose some ability to respond to antigens they had not before encountered. The findings have yet to be confirmed by others.

Studies in space of the immune system are intended to help predict impacts on health in the years ahead, when many people will have reasons for trips off this planet. But they will also provide new insights into the ordinary workings of the immune systems of earthbound mortals.

Meanwhile, on earth, research into the immune system moves ahead at such a pace that the majority of us find it difficult to keep informed. For researchers, the biggest recent breakthrough was the discovery of T cell receptors, the molecules T cells wear that read "I am a T cell" and by which they identify antigens. Scientists had been searching for this receptor non-stop for more than a decade when it was identified in 1984 by Dr. Tak Mak and colleagues at the Ontario Cancer Institute in Toronto, who found the human T cell receptor, and almost simultaneously by Dr. Mark Davis at Stanford University, who identified the mouse counterpart.

In 1986, two other groups of scientists, at Columbia University in New York and the Dana Farber Cancer Institute in Boston, reported at the Sixth International Congress on Immunology, held in Toronto, they had discovered a second T cell receptor; it is found on certain T cells that don't carry the receptor found by Dr. Tak and Dr.

Davis. Although it is too early to predict its importance, scientists hailed it as a new window into the T cell through which they hope to learn more.

The first T cell receptor, the most important one, is considered a bridge over a major gap in knowledge about the body's defense mechanisms. Until it was discovered, scientists had no direct way of finding out how T cells recognize an antigen and how they then order B cells to make antibodies. Researchers already have learned that the genes in a T cell, which tell the cell how to make a T cell receptor, can shuffle themselves around to produce a variety of receptor proteins. Consequently, the receptor can be altered to detect new antigens. The discovery has opened the door to all kinds of research. Many diseases, such as arthritis and multiple sclerosis, are the result of disorders of T cells. Now there is a way to probe T cells to find out what has gone wrong.

Other investigators are digging into the genes that control the ability of the immune system to recognize that cells in transplanted organs are foreign. They are known as the major histocompatibility complex, composed of human leukocyte antigen (HLA) genes. Scientists are just beginning to find out how many things in the body these genes govern. For example, in mice, those mouse genes control even the individual odor of a species. Mice tend to prefer as a mate a mouse whose HLA genes (in mice they are called H-2) are different. It may be nature's method of preventing a species from becoming too inbred. The mouse can smell the difference. More than ten years ago, long before this was proven, the delightful and often whimsical scientist–author, Dr. Lewis Thomas, predicted that tracking dogs could be trained to perceive HLA types in man. People with matching HLAs are compatible as donor and recipient in transplants. Not that doctors have plans to use blood-hounds to match tissues for transplants, but it gives you an idea of how far-reaching and all-important those HLA genes may be to our behavior as well as our health.

It is known that people with certain patterns of HLA genes are more prone to developing particular kinds of auto-immune diseases. We can expect much information that may prove helpful in the treatment of these diseases to be forthcoming. If, for example, doctors know that people with a particular pattern of HLA genes will, under certain circumstances — such as encountering a specific virus — develop one kind of auto-immune disease, vaccines specifically designed for high-risk groups could prevent them from being infected with that virus. Within a decade, it is likely that the culprits playing a role in many auto-immune diseases — viruses or other factors — will have been identified.

In the near future a permanent remedy for one type of inherited immune deficiency is expected to become available. The cure involves genetic engineering.

The cause of this form of immune deficiency is lack of genes that code for an enzyme called adenosine deaminase. Using a virus, scientists at Toronto's Mount Sinai Research Institute and the Hospital for Sick Children may be able to insert those missing genes into bone marrow cells of patients. They would replace the viral genes with enzyme genes and then "infect" the bone marrow. Infected stem cells in the bone marrow (from which blood cells originate) would, henceforth produce the enzyme. The virus, of course, without its own genes, is no longer a threat to health. The researchers have shown that the techniques works in animals.

Hot topics for research are the substances immune cells produce such as interleukin and interferon. Already they are being tried in treatment for different kinds of diseases. But more of them are being discovered and studied all the time — for example, substances that suppressor cells send out to slow down the immune response and, on the other side of the scale, substances that help fight the battle. One group of small proteins, discovered recently, is produced by white cells called neutrophils. Scientists call the substances "defensins" because they help defend against bacteria, fungi, and several viruses; they are almost like antibiotics, although quite distinct from any known antibiotic drugs. Scientists are now learning to make copies of them in the laboratory in hope they might be useful for some kinds of therapy.

Scientists may not yet know all the kinds of warrior cells that exist in the immune system. Not long ago, at the University of North Carolina, researchers found a new tiny cell, an off-shoot of the normal neutrophil, but much smaller. They speculate that it might be able to get into areas in which germs can be hiding but that the ordinary neutrophil can't reach. Previously unknown substances that immune cells produce are also under study. We've learned much in previous chapters about interleukin-1 and 2. Interleukin-3 has also been identified in mice and found to promote growth of some immune cells, although little is understood about its role as yet. Interleukin-4a, discovered in 1986 at the Dana Farber Cancer Institute in Boston, is believed to be able to call to battle even T cells not programmed to recognize a particular enemy. Ordinarily, immune cells only go into combat when they recognize one specific antigen.

Wound healing is still another area of investigation that is revealing more about the immune system. Macrophages, for instance, are essential for normal healing. They clean away damaged tissue and eat any foreign particles or infectious organisms that might be in the wound. But now scientists have found that macrophages are also vital in providing a new supply of oxygen to the injured tissue. In tissue deprived of oxygen, macrophages secrete a factor that stimulates the growth of tiny blood vessels. That finding may lead to a new way of controlling the growth of cancer. Many rapidly growing tumors are known to be short of oxygen at the central core, where there is a lack of circulation. Without oxygen from the blood, the center of the tumor would die, but the tumor cells usually manage to get a network of new blood vessels. Macrophages, often present in fairly large numbers in tumors, may unwittingly help them get this nourishment pipeline. New ways to stop the growth of blood vessels in tumors, so they will starve, are under study. A number of other natural products in the body have been found to play roles in formation of new blood vessels.

Macrophages may also play a role in heart disease. They produce interleukin-1, which indirectly acts on the walls of blood vessels, and doctors are investigating ways of modifying this action to prevent blood clots.

Natural killer cells are the focus of still other studies. They patrol continuously on search and destroy missions and can kill tumor cells. At Queen's University in Kingston, Ontario, scientists have found that in mice, low levels of natural killer cells correspond to the development of more tumors. Further studies are aimed at finding out how natural killer cells recognize tumor cells. They don't need T cells to tell them. But if natural killer cells can "see" something, possibly a sugar molecule, on a tumor cell, which is a tip-off that the cell is malignant, maybe doctors can learn to detect it, too. It would then be possible, some day, to make a sort of vaccine with which to show the tumor molecule to the immune system, spurring the system to be prepared for any future appearance of the molecule.

In lung cancers, doctors have found that tumors produce a substance that stimulates the cells' own growth. At the U.S. National Cancer Institute, scientists plan to give antibodies made in the laboratory against the growth substance, to patients with otherwise untreatable small-cell lung cancer. They call the antibody injection material "anti-bombesin."

Research into AIDS has disclosed that the AIDS virus gains entry to a T helper cell, the cell that has been called the conductor of the immune orchestra, by means of the cell's receptor, the molecule that identifies the cell as a T helper, also called a T4 cell. (The receptor is described earlier in this chapter.) In the laboratory, researchers have made antibodies to parts of the T4 receptor which block docking sites the virus would use to take hold of the cell when it drifts alongside — much as a spacecraft docks at a satellite station. The finding has raised hope that such antibodies might be used to prevent AIDS from developing in people exposed to the virus, or even as a vaccine, to be given to people who belong to groups at high risk of getting AIDS. The aim is to stop the AIDS virus from gaining entry to T helper cells.

Doctors at the U.S. National Cancer Institute have found that a majority of AIDS patients have high levels of one of the hormones made by the thymus gland. The finding was unexpected because levels of the hormone are abnormally low in children with inherited immune deficiencies. The hormone stimulates production of interleukin-2, revving up reproduction of T cells. But in AIDS patients, it may simply increase the numbers of T cells the AIDS virus infects. Antibodies to the hormone may help fight the disease.

Doctors suspect that some diseases with previously unknown causes may be immune system diseases. Some kinds of ulcers of the digestive tract and some skin diseases, such as psoriasis, are under investigation. One day that might mean totally new approaches to treatment for a number of ailments that are difficult to cure today.

Other researchers have found a link between certain genes in cells, called oncogenes, and auto-immune diseases, such as lupus. Oncogenes, discovered in recent years, were thought to be connected only with cancer. In healthy cells, these genes regulate other genes. In cancer, they seem to pour out proteins that cause tumor growth. In auto-immune diseases, they don't do that but may have got their messages crossed and make mistakes in the regulation of other genes. Some scientists have suggested that it might be possible in future to shut off a gene that is making mistakes by using genetic "masking tape." They might insert a phony component into the gene so that its instructions could not be read by the other genes that it regulates.

New drugs that affect only one part of the immune system, instead of shutting down the whole network, are certain to appear in coming years. Cyclosporine A, the drug that has proven invaluable in transplants and is now being tested as a treatment for auto-immune diseases, was the first one. It demonstrated that it was possible to silence certain T cells without leaving patients bereft of any defenses. Better ones, less toxic that cyclosporine A, are on the drawing board. As mentioned in Chapter Three, Japanese scientists have already announced they have devised one. So have Australian researchers. Other drugs that boost the activity of immune cells are also being designed and some are already being used in attempts to help prevent infections in patients, for instance cancer patients whose immune systems have been suppressed by cancer drugs or radio-therapy, and in AIDS patients.

Most exciting to some scientists are the tantalizing new findings about connections between the brain, many hormones in the body, and the immune system. One of the latest discoveries is a connection between T cells and prolactin (a hormone produced by the pituitary gland whose only previously known function was in production of breast milk). If the hormone is blocked out of T cells, they stop producing interleukin-2. Every such discovery raises many questions, stimulating more research to find the answers. Some immunologists predict that eventually it will be possible to remedy problems in the immune system, replacing substances that are lacking, just as today doctors can treat deficiencies in the endocrine (hormone) system — for example, by giving essential homones at a time of stress, such as surgery, to patients deficient in certain hormones needed to cope with stress. Before that was possible, surgery was often life-threatening to such people.

"Today, it is as if (scientists) are looking down at the immune system as if we were observing earth from a satellite," says the University of Western Ontario's Dr. Calvin Stiller. "We can see troops and planes move from country to country. We send spies out (investigational studies) and they come back and we think we gain insight into why the troops are moving. But there is a whole series of movements we don't understand. We can't see, from the satellite, that there are commands from high levels, possibly a kind of United Nations, to which the troops are responding. We have not yet tapped into an information network at a second level, where the immune system is integrated with hormones and nerves. The way in which those connections are made at a molecular level is yet to be defined."

When it is defined, it will revolutionize medical care.

Overall, the amount of research into the immune system is enormous. What has been described is only a sample. One thing, however, is quite clear. Man may have achieved marvellously complex technology that can take us to the moon and give us computers that can see and think. But man has come nowhere near building a system as exquisitely complicated as the immune system within you. As with any system composed of a multitude of components and controls, sometimes things can go wrong. A part becomes flawed or a crack appears. The miracle is that the immune system works so beautifully, its parts operating in incredible harmony, most of the time.

Some day, when scientists have brought together all the pieces and solved the many mysteries that remain, doctors will know how to repair any breakdowns. Many diseases that today seem incurable will no longer plague us. That will be the happy ending of the immune system story you will read some day. For now, this book must remain like a detective novel with the final chapters missing. Keep tuned to tomorrow; eventually the mysteries will be solved.

GLOSSARY

AIDS: acquired immune deficiency syndrome: a fatal disease caused by a virus that infects key immune cells.

ALLERGEN: a substance, such as pollen, dust, or animal dander, that can cause an allergic reaction.

ALLERGIC REACTION: an adverse reaction made by the immune system to otherwise harmless substances.

ALLOGRAFT: transplant of tissue from donor other than an identical twin.

ANAPHYLAXIS: a severe allergic reaction that can cause shock and collapse.

ANGIOEDEMA: a reaction in the skin and underlying tissue involving redness and swelling.

ANTIBODY: a Y-shaped protein produced by certain cells of the immune system as one line of defense against germs. Antibodies are also called immunoglobulins.

ANTIGEN: a molecule, formed of protein and carbohydrates, of a cell or other organism such as a virus, against which an immune response can be made.

ARC: AIDS-related complex: a syndrome involving some symptoms typical of acquired immune deficiency syndrome (AIDS) which can, but does not always, develop into full-blown AIDS.

ARV: AIDS-related virus. A virus similar to, but not identical with, the virus that causes AIDS.

ATOPIC: having an inherited tendency to develop allergy.

AUTO-ANTIBODY: an antibody produced against ordinary tissue in a person's own body.

BACTERIA: one-celled organisms containing genetic material, DNA or RNA, and cellular material. Of the hundreds of different types, a few cause serious diseases in humans.

BASOPHIL: a white blood cell, similar to mast cells, which releases histamine and other compounds involved in allergic reactions.

B CELL: a white cell that produces antibodies.

BLOCKING ANTIBODY: antibody that protects against damage by other antibodies and immune cells by blocking their attack. Also called enhancing antibody.

BONE MARROW: soft tissue within bones where blood cells originate.

BRONCHIOLE: tiny airway that is part of the tree-like network of airways in each lung.

BRONCHODILATOR: drug used to relax smooth muscles in airways, often used to treat acute asthma.

BRONCHOSPASM: tightening of the muscles around airway tubes.

CEA: carcinoembryonic antigen; a substance produced naturally before birth but only found in adults in connection with certain diseases including some cancers.

CELL-MEDIATED IMMUNITY: line of defense involved in attacking infected cells of the body or foreign cells, such as those in transplanted tissue.

CHALLENGE TEST: a test to identify substances to which a person is sensitive or allergic by exposing the person to tiny amounts of such substances.

CHEMOTACTIC FACTORS: chemicals released in the body to attract immune cells to the site of an infection or inflammation.

COMBINED IMMUNE DEFICIENCY SYNDROME: a condition in which a person lacks both lines of body defenses.

COMPLEMENT: a family of proteins in the blood that works with antibodies to destroy infected or foreign cells.

CYCLOSPORINE A: a drug that suppresses one part of the cell-mediated immune system and is used to prevent rejection of transplanted organs. Also being tested against auto-immune diseases.

CYTOTOXIC: destructive to cells.

DANDER: small scales from animal skin, a common allergen.

DELAYED-TYPE HYPERSENSITIVITY: a slow immune response caused by immune cells, but not by antibodies.

DERMATITIS: inflammation of the skin. Contact dermatitis may be an allergic rash caused by allergens touching the skin.

DIABETES: a condition in which insulin produced by the pancreas is lacking or unable to keep blood sugar levels in balance. Type I diabetes is believed to be an auto-immune disease in which cells that produce insulin are destroyed.

DI GEORGE SYNDROME: an immune deficiency condition that is inherited.

DNA: deoxyribonucleic acid, genetic material that carries the instructions for life processes and is contained by every cell in the body.

ECZEMA: a non-contagious, itching, sometimes weeping, inflammation of the skin.

ELISA: enzyme-linked immunosorbent assay. A laboratory test used to look for antibodies against certain diseases, including AIDS.

EDEMA: abnormal pool of fluid in tissue.

ENDOTOXIN: a cell wall component shed by some bacteria that can generate a strong immune response.

ENHANCING ANTIBODY: see blocking antibody.

EOSINOPHIL: a type of white blood cell that plays a part in immune responses.

EXOTOXIN: substance given off by bacteria that can damage cells or tissue.

FACTOR VIII: clotting factor in blood lacking in people with common form of hemophilia; is given them as a blood product obtained from pooled blood of several thousand donors.

FLARE: redness on the skin around an elevated area called a wheal, often indicating an allergic reaction.

FOOD ALLERGY: a reaction to certain foods that may show up as severe indigestion, diarrhea, skin rash, or breathing problems.

FUNGI: organisms usually made up of more than one cell, resembling plants but lacking chlorophyll; hence they must live off other forms of life or dead matter. Of thousands of types of fungi, about 10 cause diseases in man.

GENE: unit of genetic material, a segment of DNA (or RNA in some organisms) carrying the code for a specific protein.

GERM: a general word for microscopic organisms that cause disease.

GRANYLOCYTE: a cell that is a member of a family of white cells containing granules that include basophils, neutrophils, and eosinophils.

GI TRACT: gastro-intestinal tract; stomach and intestines.

HAPTEN: a molecule that does not, by itself, cause an immune reaction, but that may be part of an antigen.

HAY FEVER: an allergic condition affecting eyes, nose, throat, and respiratory tract; also called allergic rhinitis.

HELPER CELL: a T cell that stimulates T cell growth, orders antibody production by B cells, and spurs macrophage activity; the conductor of the immune cell orchestra.

HISTAMINE: a chemical released by mast cells, responsible for much of the itching, swelling, and congestion typical of allergies.

HISTOCOMPATIBILITY: a measure of tissue similarity of two individuals. Histocompatibility antigens are molecules that immune cells recognize as "self" or "foreign" markers and are involved in rejection of a transplanted organ.

HIVES: raised, itchy patches on the skin. Also called wheals or urticaria.

HLA: human leukocyte antigens. Markers on cells that identify an individual as unique. Only identical twins have the same HLA.

Body Defenses

HTLV III: human T cell lymphotropic virus, type three; HTLV I and HTLV II cause certain kinds of cancer. HTLV III is the cause of AIDS. The same virus is also called LAV, for lymphadenopathy-associated virus. A name widely used combines the two — LAV/HTLV III — but a simpler name, HIV, for human immune-deficiency virus, has been accepted internationally.

HUMORAL IMMUNITY: the arm of defense involving B cells, antibodies, and complement.

IDIOTYPE: segment on an antibody that fits a precise antigen structure.

IMMUNE COMPLEX: antibody and antigen bound together.

IMMUNOGLOBULIN: antibodies; a family of proteins.

INTERFERON: a family of chemicals produced by cells in response to infection to stimulate body defenses.

INTERLEUKINS: hormones produced by immune cells. Interleukin-1 is produced by macrophages; interleukin-2, a growth factor, is produced by T cells. Immune cells communicate by means of interleukins.

ISLET CELLS: cells in the pancreas that produce insulin; also called Beta cells.

JUVENILE DIABETES: also called type I; the kind of diabetes believed to be an auto-immune disease.

JOINT: connections between bones, such as juncture in knee or elbow, common sites affected by arthritis.

KAPOSI'S SARCOMA: form of rare cancer that occurs in patients with AIDS.

KILLER CELLS: members of the T cell family that destroy infected cells and cancer cells.

LAV: see HTLV; virus believed to cause AIDS.

LEUKOCYTES: also spelled leucocytes, all white blood cells, of which there are five classifications.

LYMPHOCYTES: one class of white blood cells that defend the body; T cells and B cells.

LYMPHADENOPATHY: a syndrome involving chronically swollen glands that may be an indication of infection with the AIDS virus.

LYMPH NODE: a small oval structure that filters lymph (yellowish fluid circulating in the lymph system) and where lymphocytes become activated. Found in the mouth, neck, armpit, groin, and elsewhere, nodes range from the size of a pinhead to a bean.

LYMPHOKINES: proteins produced by lymphocytes for communication; chemical signals governing the immune response.

LUPUS: systemic lupus erythematosus; an auto-immune disease, damaging many body systems; particularly affecting blood vessels and kidneys.

MACROPHAGE: a large white blood cell, vital to body defense; a member of a white cell family called monocytes; garbage collector for the bloodstream.

MAST CELLS: cells in tissue that contain packets of chemicals, such as histamine, responsible for symptoms of allergy.

MEMORY CELL: a long-lived T or B cell that recognizes a particular antigen that has been in the body before; the key to immunization.

MICROBE: a microscopic disease-causing organism; may be a virus, bacterium, or fungus.

MONOCLONAL ANTIBODIES: antibodies produced by specially created identical cells (clone); the cells can be primed to produce any one specific type of antibody.

MOLD: microscopic, spore-producing plants, sometimes involved in allergies.

MULTIPLE SCLEROSIS: often shortened to MS, a condition in which insulating sheaths of nerves are damaged; believed to be an auto-immune disease.

MYASTHENIA GRAVIS: a condition characterized by weakness of muscles; an auto-immune disease.

MYELIN: the sheath covering nerves, affected by MS.

NATURAL KILLER CELL: a white cell, cousin of T cells, that attacks virus-infected cells and cancer cells.

NEUTROPHIL: grain-like white cell, involved in destroying and removing bacteria; blood levels of neutrophils rise as a result of sudden infection.

ONCOLOGY: the study of cancer.

ONCOGENE: a gene, usually governing cell growth, it may, under certain conditions, make cancer grow.

OPPORTUNISTIC INFECTIONS: caused by germs, generally not harmful to normal people but that take advantage of weakened body defenses to cause serious disease.

PATHOGEN: a disease-causing micro-organism; may be a virus, bacterium or fungus.

PHAGOCYTE: cell that engulfs (eats) pathogens or other foreign particles; may be a macrophage or granulocyte.

PROSTAGLANDIN: a hormone-like fatty acid; different ones have different effects and act on muscles or certain organs.

PROTOZOA: one-celled organisms that move by means of flagella; one kind of protozoa causes malaria.

Q FEVER: a feverish illness, caused by an organism (rickettsia), which is contracted from infected cattle or sheep; vaccination against Q fever is recommended for people working with domestic animals.

RETROVIRUS: a sub-species of virus equipped with an enzyme (reverse transcriptase), with which viral genetic material can be inserted into the DNA of a cell; the AIDS virus and cancer viruses are retroviruses.

RHINITIS: inflammation of the membrane lining the nose.

RNA: ribonucleic acid, genetic material of retroviruses.

REJECTION: an attack by immune cells on transplanted tissue.

SCID: severe combined immune deficiency; an inborn defect of both humoral and cell-mediated immunity.

SCLERODERMA: a rare disease affecting blood vessels and connective tissue, considered an auto-immune disease.

SENSITIVITY: increased reaction to substances that are harmless to people without allergies.

SUPPRESSOR CELLS: a sub-set of T cells that bring an immune response to an end.

T CELLS: white cells (lymphocytes) that provide cell-mediated immunity; certain T cells are the commanders of the immune system.

THYMUS: organ of the immune system in which T cells mature.

TISSUE MATCHING: tests to determine the compatibility of donor and recipient, done prior to transplantation.

TUMOR NECROSIS FACTOR: a lymphokine that may help destroy tumors.

UNIVERSAL REACTOR: a person who suffers adverse reactions to many environmental substances.

URTICARIA: hives; a reaction in skin with swelling, redness, and itching.

VACCINE: a substance containing antigens to disease-causing organisms that will bring about a protective immune response.

VIRUS: a microscopic germ, which causes disease by invading cells, forcing them to become virus manufacturers; different viruses cause a wide array of diseases from the common cold to AIDS.

WESTERN BLOT: a laboratory test used to detect antibodies, for example, antibodies to AIDS.

WHEAL: an elevation of the skin, often itchy, such as caused by an insect bite or an allergen.

XENOGRAFT: transplanted tissue from another species.

YEAST: a fungus; candida albicans is one kind of disease-producing yeast.

ZOSTER IMMUNE GLOBULIN: an antibody-containing drug, used in immune-deficient patients to combat herpes zoster (shingles), a painful infection causing blisters on the skin overlying nerve pathways.

DIRECTORY

Where to find help

AIDS:

United States:

AIDS Action Council
Federation of AIDS-Related
Organizations
1115½ Independence Ave. SE
Washington, D.C. 20003

AIDS Medical Foundation
10 E. 13th St.
New York, NY 10003

Gay Rights National Lobby
P.O. Box 1892
Washington, D.C. 20013

National Gay Task Force
80 Fifth Ave., Ste. 1601
New York, NY 10011

Haitian Coalition on AIDS
255 Eastern Pkwy. Apt. 2A
Brooklyn, NY 11238

Canada:

NAC-AIDS
Laboratory Centre for
Disease Control
Health and Welfare Canada
Ottawa, Ont. K1A 8N8

AIDS Vancouver
1033 Davie St.,
Ste. 308
Vancouver, B.C. V6E 1M7

AIDS Committee of Toronto
P.O. Box 55, Stn. F
Toronto, Ont. M4Y 2L4

Comite SIDA Aide Montreal
C.P. 98, Depot N
Montreal, Que. H2X 3M2

Booklets available:

Facts on Aids for the public
($7.95)
The Canadian Public Health
Association
1335 Carling Ave., Ste. 210
Ottawa, Ont. K1Z 8N8

Answers About AIDS ($2.00)
A report by the American Council on
Science and Health
47 Maple St.
Summit, NJ 07901

ALLERGY:

United States:

American Academy of
Allergy and Immunology
611 E. Wells St.
Milwaukee, WI 53202

Asthma and Allergy Foundation
of America
1302 18th St. NW, Ste. 303
Washington, D.C. 20036

American Allergy Association
P.O. Box 7273
Menico Park, CA 94026

<u>Canada:</u>

Allergy Information
Association
Room 7, 25 Poynter Dr.
Weston, Ont. M9R 1K8

Canadian Lung Association
75 Albert St., Ste. 908
Ottawa, Ont. K1P 5E7

ARTHRITIS:

Arthritis Society of Canada
250 Bloor St. E., Ste. 401
Toronto, Ont. M4W 3P2

National Arthritis and
Musculoskeletal and Skin
Diseases Information
Clearinghouse,
P.O. Box 9782
Arlington, VA 22209

Arthritis Foundation
3400 Peachtree Rd. NE
Atlanta, GA 30326

CANCER:

American Cancer Society
777 Third Avenue
New York, NY 10017

Canadian Cancer Society
77 Bloor St., Ste. 1702
Toronto, Ont. M5S 3A1

DIABETES:

American Diabetes Association
2 Park Avenue
New York, NY 10016

Juvenile Diabetes Foundation
International
60 Madison Ave.
New York, NY 10010

Canadian Diabetes Association
123 Edward St., Ste. 601
Toronto, Ont. M5G 1E2

Juvenile Diabetes Research
Foundation
4632 Yonge St., Ste. 201
Willowdale, Ont. M2N 5M1

MULTIPLE SCLEROSIS:

Multiple Sclerosis Society
of Canada
250 Bloor St. E., Ste. 820
Toronto, Ont. M4W 3P9

National MS Society
205 E. 42nd St.
New York, NY 10017

MYASTHENIA GRAVIS:

Myasthenia Gravis Foundation
15 E. 26th St., Ste. 1603
New York, NY 10010

TRANSPLANTS:

Organ Recovery
1991 Lee Rd.
Cleveland Heights, OH 44118

Transplant International
399 Windermere Rd.
London, Ont. N6A 5A5

American Heart Association
7320 Greenville Ave.
Dallas, TX 75231

Canadian Heart Foundation
1 Nicholas St., Ste. 1200
Ottawa, Ont. K1N 7B7

National Kidney Foundation
2 Park Ave.
New York, NY 10016

Kidney Foundation of Canada
1650 De Maisonneuve Blvd. W.
Ste. 400
Montreal, Que. H3H 2P3

National Association of Patients
on Hemodialysis and
Transplantation
156 William St.
New York, NY 10038

American Liver Foundation
998 Pompton Ave.
Cedar Grove, NJ 07009

Canadian Liver Foundation
42 Charles St. E., Ste. 510
Toronto, Ont. M4Y 1T4

VACCINES AND INFECTIOUS DISEASES:

American Academy of Pediatrics
141 Northwest Point Rd.
P.O. Box 927
Elk Grove Village, IL 60007

National Foundation for
Infectious Diseases
P.O. Box 42022
Washington, D.C. 20015

Canadian Pediatric Society
Children's Hospital of
Eastern Ontario
401 Smyth Rd.
Ottawa, Ont. K1H 8L1